LECTURES

ON

HOMŒOPATHIC
PHILOSOPHY

BY

JAMES TYLER KENT, A.M., M.D.

AUTHOR OF REPERTORY OF THE HOMŒOPATHIC MATERIA MEDICA,
AND LECTURES ON HOMŒOPATHIC MATERIA MEDICA, ETC. DEAN
OF THE POST GRADUATE SCHOOL OF HOMŒOPATHY IN
PHILADELPHIA FOR NINE YEARS. PROFESSOR OF
MATERIA MEDICA AT HAHNEMANN MEDICAL COL-
LEGE AND HOSPITAL IN CHICAGO FOR SIX
YEARS, AND OF THE HERING MEDICAL
COLLEGE IN CHICAGO FOR SOME
YEARS AFTER.

North Atlantic Books
Homeopathic Educational Services
Berkeley, California

Lectures on Homoeopathic Philosophy
by James Tyler Kent

ISBN 0–913028–61–4

Originally published in 1900

Foreword © 1979 by Dana Ullman, M.P.H.

Publishers' Addresses:

North Atlantic Books
P.O. Box 12327
Berkeley, California 94712

Homeopathic Educational Services
2124 Kittredge Street
Berkeley, California 94705

Cover design: Paula Morrison

Lectures on Homoeopathic Philosophy is sponsored by the Society for the Study of Native Arts and Sciences, a nonprofit educational corporation whose goals are to develop an educational and crosscultural perspective linking various scientific, social, and artistic fields; to nurture a holistic view of arts, sciences, humanities, and healing; and to publish and distribute literature on the relationship of mind, body, and nature.

North Atlantic Books' publications are available through most bookstores. For further information, call 800-337-2665 or visit our website at: www.northatlanticbooks.com.

Substantial discounts on bulk quantities are available to corporations, professional associations, and other organizations. For details and discount information, contact our special sales department.

---

4 5 6 7 8 9 / 08 07 06 05 04 03 02

Foreword to the New Edition

Lectures on Homoeopathic Philosophy is one of three books by Dr. James Tyler Kent, all of which are classics in the homoeopathic literature. In this book Dr. Kent summarizes, interprets, and systematizes Samuel Hahnemann's treatise of homoeopathy *The Organon of the Healing Art*. This is the first book to synthesize comprehensively the writings of Hahnemann and the traditions of classical homoeopathy. As such, *Lectures on Homoeopathic Philosophy* is must reading for any student or practitioner of homoeopathy as well as any individual seriously interested in understanding fundamental laws of health and healing.

When Dr. Kent wrote this book at the turn of the twentieth century, homoeopathy was near its peak of popularity in the United States. There were eighteen homoeopathic medical schools, at least one hundred homoeopathic hospitals, and more than one thousand pharmacies carrying homoeopathic remedies. During this time, between twenty and twenty-five percent of the practicing physicians in urban areas considered themselves homoeopaths.

Despite their great numbers, Kent was dissatisfied with the quality of homoeopathic practice. Most of these physicians utilized the homoeopathic remedies in a mechanistic and reductionistic manner similar to the way in which orthodox physicians prescribed drugs. Frequently, these "homocopaths" violated many basic tenets of classical homoeopathy by prescribing more than one remedy at a time, by recommending frequent repetition of doses, and by prescribing a remedy based upon a person's disease rather than his or her individualized symptoms.

Kent re-establishes the philosophical basis of classical homoeopathy and elaborates the structure and methodology of Hahnemannian thought. This book was his ardent commitment to the resurrection of the classical Hahnemannian traditions. However, the active economic and legal oppression against the homoeopaths by orthodox physicians left Kent in an uphill and losing position even as he wrote. Furthermore, he was articulating an empirical, vitalistic medicine at a time when many homoeopaths were adopting the more rational physicobiochemic approach of the mainstream science.

Kent was unambiguously an empirical Hahnemannian. In some portions of this book, he offers sharp criticism of pseudo-homoeopaths and their rationalist practices, while other portions critique the often treacherous treatments of orthodox medicine in 1900. Although the harshness of his criticism must be understood in the context of his time, the reader will find much of his criticism of both homoeopathic and orthodox medical practice still relevant today.

Even though this book was written approximately eighty years ago, the concepts of health and healing still remain ahead of our time. Insights into the essential characteristics of the healing process are found throughout this book. Kent describes how to take a person's case history, how to study the case, how to establish the hierarchy of symptoms in determining the appropriate remedy, and above all, how to decide what to do after the first prescription, how to interpret the many reactions following its actions, and how scientifically to understand what is a cure.

Homoeopathy is a particularly relevant health practice today, considering our new knowledge in quantum physics, immunology, epidemiology, holistic health, and other fields of natural and social science. New fields of study today begin to echo the concepts that Kent elucidates in this book.

The following quotes show the range and depth of Kent's thought:

"The whole aim of the physician is to secure the language of nature. If it has been masked by medicine, it cannot be secured."

"There is no disease that exists of which the cause is known to man by the eye or by the microscope. Causes are infinitely too fine to be observed by any instrument of precision. They are so immaterial that they correspond to and operate upon the interior nature of man, and they are ultimated in the body in form of tissue changes that are recognized by the eye. Such tissue changes must be understood as the results of disease only or the physician will never perceive what disease cause is, what disease is, what potentization is, or what the nature of life is."

"Susceptibility is only a name for a state that underlies all possible sickness and all possible cure."

"Do not say that the patient is sick because he has a white swelling, but that the white swelling is there because the patient is sick."

Dr. Kent is also the author of two other indispensable books in homoeopathy. Kent's *Repertory of the Homoeopathic Materia Medica* is the most comprehensive and reliable compendium of the symptoms in homoeopathy. In its 1423 pages, various homoeopathic remedies are listed by symptom, based upon the tendency of the remedy to cause and thus cure the symptoms. *Lectures on the Homoeopathic Materia Medica* is another classic of homoeopathic literature. It complements the *Repertory* by describing the specific "psycho-physiologic personalities" of 180 homoeopathic remedies. The proper use of these books is described in Kent's *Lectures on Homoeopathic Philosophy*.

James Tyler Kent's *Lectures on Homoeopathic Philosophy* is an excellent book to start one's study of homoeopathy, and ultimately an important book to re-read throughout one's involvement in the healing arts.

—*Dana Ullman, M.P.H.*

For Further Study in Homeopathic Medicine

INTRODUCTORY AND SELF-HELP BOOKS:

Everybody's Guide to Homeopathic Medicine, Stephen Cummings, M.D., and Dana Ullman, M.P.H.
Homeopathy: An Introduction for Beginners and Skeptics, Richard Grossinger
The Homeopathic Emergency Guide, Thomas Kruzel, N.D.
The Consumer's Guide to Homeopathy, Dana Ullman, M.P.H.
Homeopathic Medicines for Children and Infants, Dana Ullman, M.P.H.
Discovering Homeopathy, Dana Ullman, M.P.H.
A Patient's Guide to Homeopathic Medicines, Robert Ullman, N.D. and Judyth Reichenberg-Ullman, N.D., M.S.W.
The Science of Homeopathy, George Vithoulkas

BOOKS FOR SERIOUS STUDENTS OR PRACTITIONERS OF HOMEOPATHY:

Homeopathy: A Frontier in Medical Science, Paolo Bellavite, M.D. and Andrea Signorini, M.D.
Divided Legacy: A History of the Schism in Medical Thought (4 volumes), Harris Coulter
The Organon of Medicine, Samuel Hahnemann, M.D.
The Spirit of Homeopathy, Rajan Sankaran
Psyche and Substance: Essays on Homeopathy in the Light of Jungian Psychology, Edward C. Whitmont, M.D.

IMPORTANT MATERIA MEDICA AND REPERTORIES

Homeopathic Psychology, Philip Bailey, M.D.
A Pocket Manual of Materia Medica with Repertory, William Boericke, M.D.
Repertory of Homeopathic Materia Medica, James T. Kent, M.D.
Desktop Guide to Keynotes and Confirmatory Symptoms, Roger Morrison, M.D.
Lotus Materia Medica, Robin Murphy, N.D.
Homeopathy and Minerals, Jan Scholten, M.D.
Synthesis Repertorium, F. Schroyens, M.D.
The Complete Repertory, Roger van Zandvoort
Concordant Materia Medica, Frans Vermeulen, M.D.

These and other books, tapes, and software are available from:

HOMEOPATHIC EDUCATIONAL SERVICES
2124 Kittredge St.
Berkeley, CA. 94704

Website: http://www.homeopathic.com

PREFACE BY DR. KENT

These lectures were delivered in the POST-GRADUATE SCHOOL OF HOMŒOPATHICS, and published in the *Journal of Homœopathics*, and, now in somewhat revised form, are given to the profession with the hope that they will prove useful to some in giving a clearer apprehension of the doctrines of Homœopathy. They are not intended, in any sense, to take the place of the *Organon*, but should be read with that work, in the form of a commentary, the object in each lecture being to dwell upon the particular doctrine sufficiently to perceive and emphasize the master's thought. Not all of the paragraphs in the *Organon* have been considered, as many of them are sufficiently clear to the reader and their teaching is quite obvious.

Homœopathy is now extensively disseminated over the world, but, strange to say, by none are its doctrines so distorted as by many of its pretended devotees. Homœopathics treats of both the *science* and the *art* of healing by the law of similars, and if the *art* is to remain and progress among men the science must be better understood than at present. To apply the art without the science is merely a pretension, and such practice should be relegated to the domain of empiricism. To safely practice the art of curing sick people, the homœopathic physician must know the science.

It is not expected that this course of lectures covers the whole field of homœopathic philosophy, but it is intended to serve as an introduction to further study, and as a text-book for students, that they may have a sound starting and become interested in the objects of this work.

JAMES TYLER KENT

Evanston, Ill., July 1, 1900

CONTENTS

LECTURES ON HOMŒOPATHIC PHILOSOPHY

LECTURE I

§ 1. "THE SICK"

Homœopathy asserts that there are *principles* which govern the practice of medicine. It may be said that, up till the time of Hahnemann, no principles of medicine were recognized, and even at this day in the writings and actions of the Old Schools there is a complete acknowledgment that no principles exist. The Old School declares that the practice of medicine depends entirely upon experience, upon what can be found out by giving medicines to the sick. Their shifting methods and theories, and rapid discoveries and abandonment of the same, fully attest the sincerity of their acknowledgments and declarations. Homœopathy leaves Allopathy at this point, and so in this manner the great division between the two schools is affected. That there are principles Homœopathy affirms. The Old School denies the existence of principles and with apparent reason, looking at the matter from the standpoint of their practice and methods. They deal only with ultimates, they observe only results of disease, and either deny or have no knowledge of the real nature of man, what he is, where he came from, what his quality is in sickness or in health. They say nothing about the man except in connection with his tissues; they characterize the changes in the tissues as the disease and all there is of the disease, its beginning and its end. In effect they proclaim disease to be something that exists without a cause. They accept nothing but what can be felt with the fingers and seen with the eyes or otherwise observed through the sense, aided by improved instruments. The finger is aided by the microscope to an elongated point, and the microscopic pathological results of disease are noted and considered to be the beginning and the ending, *i.e.* results without anything prior to them. That is a summary of allopathic teaching as to the nature of sickness. But Homœopathy perceives that there is something prior to these results. Every science teaches, and every investigation of a scientific character proves that everything which exists does so because of something prior to it. Only in this way can we trace cause and effect in a series from beginning to end and back again from the end to the beginning. By this means we arrive at a state in which we do not assume, but in which we know.

The first paragraph of the *Organon* will be understood by an inexperienced observer to mean one thing and by a true and experienced homœopath to mean another.

§ 1. "The physician's high and *only* mission is to restore the sick to health, to cure as it is termed."

No controversy will arise from a superficial reading of this state-ment, and until Hahnemann's hidden meaning of the word "sick" is fully brought to view, the physician of any school will assent. The idea that one person will entertain as to the meaning of the word "sick" will be different at times from that which another will enter-tain. So long as it remains a matter of opinion, there will be differ-ences of opinion, therefore the homœopath must abandon the mere expressions of opinion. Allopathy rests on individual opinion and allopaths say that the science of medicine is based on the consensus of opinion, but that is an unworthy and unstable foundation for the science of curing the sick. It will never be possible to establish a rational system of therapeutics until we reason from facts as they are and not as they sometimes appear. Facts as they appear are ex-pressed in the opinions of men, but facts as they are, are facts and truths from which doctrines are evolved and formulated which will interpret or unlock the kingdoms of nature in the realm of sickness or health. Therefore, beware of the opinion of men in science. Hahnemann has given us principles which we can study and advance upon. It is law that governs the world and not matters of opinion or hypotheses. We must begin by having a respect for law, for we have no starting point unless we base our propositions on law. So long as we recognize men's statements we are in a state of change, for men and hypotheses change. Let us acknowledge the authority.

The true homœopath, when he speaks of *the sick*, knows who it is that is sick, whereas the allopath does not know. The latter thinks that the house which the man lives in, which is being torn down, expresses all there is of sickness; in other words, that the tissue changes (which are only the *results* of disease) are all that there is of the sick man. The homœopath observes wonderful changes resulting from potentized medicine, and being compelled to reflect he sees that crude drugs cannot heal the sick and that what changes they do effect are not real but only apparent. Modern physiology has no vital doctrine in its teaching, and therefore no basis to work upon. The doctrine of the vital force is not admitted by the teachers of physiology and, therefore, the homœopath sees that true physiology is not yet taught, for without the vital force, without simple substance, without the internal as well as the external, there can be no *cause* and no relation between cause and effect.

Now what is meant by "the sick?" It is a man that is sick and to be restored to health, not his body, not the issues. You will find many people who will say, "I am sick." They will enumerate pages of symptoms, pages of suffering. They look sick. But they tell you, "I have been to the most eminent physicians. I have had my chest examined. I have been to the neurologist. I have been to the cardiac specialist and have had my heart examined. The eye specialist has examined my eyes. I have been to the gynæcologist and have had my uterus examined", says the woman. "I have been physically examined from head to foot, and they tell me I am not sick, I have no disease." Many a time have I heard this story after getting three or four pages of symptoms. What does it mean? It is true if that state progresses there will *be* evidences of disease, *i.e.*, evidences which the pathologist may discover by his physical examination. But at present the patient is not sick, says the learned doctor, "But what do all these symptoms mean? I do not sleep at night. I have pains and aches. My bowels do not move."

"Oh, well, you have constipation." That is the first thing that has been diagnosed. But do all these things exist without a cause? It would seem from one opinion that the "constipation" is the disease *per se*, but from another opinion it would appear to be the cause of disease; the "diagnosis" is made to apply to one as much as to the other. But this is the character of vagaries so common to Old School whims. These symptoms are but the language of nature, talking out as it were, and showing as clearly as the daylight the internal nature of the sick man or woman. If this state progresses the lungs break down. The doctor says, "Oh, now you have consumption;" or a great change appears in the liver, and he says, "Oh, now you have fatty degeneration of the liver;" or albumen appears in the urine, and he tells the patient, "Now I am able to name your disease. You have some one of the forms of Bright's disease." It is nonsense to say that prior to the localization of disease, the patient is not sick. Does it not seem clear that this patient has been sick, and very sick, even from childhood? Under traditional methods it is necessary that a diagnosis be made before the treatment can be settled, but in most cases the diagnosis cannot be made until the results of disease have rendered the patient incurable.

Again, take the nervous child. It has wild dreams, twitching, restless sleep, nervous excitement, hysterical manifestations, but if we examine all the organs of the body we will find nothing the matter with them. This sickness, however, which is present, if allowed to go on uncured, will in twenty or thirty years result in tissue change; the organs will become affected and then it will be said that the body is diseased; but the individual has been sick from the beginning. It is a question whether we will start out and consider the results of disease or begin at the beginning with the causes. If we have material ideas of disease we will have material ideas of the means of cure. If we believe an organ is sick and alone constitutes the disease, we must feel that if we could remove the organ we would cure the patient. A man has a necrotic condition of the hand; then if we believe that only the hand is sick we would think we had cured the patient by removing his hand. Say the hand is cancerous. According to this idea it is cancerous in itself and from itself, and seeing he would later die from the cancer of his hand we would conscientiously remove the hand and so cure the patient. For an eruption on the skin we would use local means to stimulate the functions of the skin and make it heal, and believing the eruption had no cause behind it we would conscientiously think we had cured the patient. But this is the *reductio ad absurdum*, for nothing exists without a cause. The organs are not the man. The man is prior to the organs. From first to last is the order of sickness as well as the order of cure. From man to his organs and not from organs to the man.

Well, then who is this sick man? The tissues could not become sick unless something prior to them had been deranged and so make them sick. What is there of this man that can be called the internal man? What is there that can be removed so that the whole that is physical may be left behind? We say that man dies but he leaves his body behind. We dissect the body and find all of his organs. Everything that we know by the senses belongs to physical man, everything that we can feel with the fingers and see with the eyes he leaves behind. The real sick man is prior to the sick body and we must conclude that the sick man be somewhere in that portion which is not left behind. That which is carried away is primary and that which is left behind is ultimate. We say the man feels, sees, tastes, hears, he thinks and he lives, but these are only outward manifestations of thinking and living. The man wills and understands; the cadaver does not will and does not understand; then that which takes its departure is that which knows and wills. It is *that* which can be changed and is prior to the body.

The combination of these two, the will and the understanding, constitute man; conjoined they make life and activity, they manufacture the body and cause all things of the body. With the will and understanding operating in order we have a healthy man. It is not our purpose to go behind the will and the understanding, to go prior to these. It is enough to say that they were created. Then man is the will and the understanding, and the house which he lives in is his body.

We must, to be scientific homœopaths, recognize that the muscles, the nerves, the ligaments and the other parts of man's frame are a picture and manifest to the intelligent physician the internal man. Both the dead and the living body are to be considered, not from the body to the life, but from the life to the body. If you were to describe the difference between two human faces, their character and everything you observe of their action, you would be describing scarcely more than the will. The will is expressed in the face; its result is implanted on the countenance. Have you ever studied the face of an individual who has grown up a murderer or villain of some sort? Is there no difference between his face and that of one who has the will to do good, to live uprightly? Go down into the lowest parts of our great city and study the faces of these people. These people are night prowlers; they are up late at night studying villainy. If we inquire into it we will see that their affections are of that kind. They have the stamp upon their faces. They have evil affections and an evil face. The countenance then is expressive of the heart. Allopathic pathology recognizes nothing but man's body. Yet one can easily confuse the allopath by asking him what man's thought is, what man is. The homœopath must master these things before he can perceive the nature of the cause of disease and before he can understand what cure is.

It is the sole duty of the physician to heal the sick. It is not his sole duty to heal the results of sickness, but the sickness itself. When the man himstlf has been restored to health, there will be restored harmony in the tissues and in the activities. Then the sole duty of the physician is to put in order the interior of the economy, i.e., the will and understanding conjoined. Tissue changes are of the body and are the results of disease. They are not the disease. Hahnemann once said, "There are no diseases, but sick people," from which it is clear that Hahnemann understood that the diseases so-called, e.g., Bright's disease, liver disease, etc. were but the grosser forms of disease results, viz., appearances of disease. There is first disorder of government, and this proceeds from within outward until we have pathological changes in the tissues. In the practice of medicine today the idea of government is not found, and the tissue changes only are taken into account.

He who considers disease results to be the disease itself, and expects to do away with these as disease, is insane. It is an insanity in medicine, an insanity that has grown out of the milder forms of mental disorder in science, crazy whims. The bacteria are results of disease. In the course of time we will be able to show perfectly that the microscopical little fellows are not the disease cause, but that they come after, that they are scavengers accompanying the disease, and that they are perfectly harmless in every respect. They are the outcome of the disease, are present wherever the disease is, and by the microscope it has been discovered that every pathological result has its corresponding bacteria. The Old School consider these the cause, but we will be able to show that disease cause is much more subtle than anything that can be shown by a microscope. We will be able to show you by a process of reasoning, step by step, the folly of hunting for disease cause by the implements of the senses.

In a note Hahnemann says: "The physician's mission is not, however, to construct so-called systems, by interweaving empty speculations and hypotheses concerning the internal essential nature of the vital processes and the mode in which diseases originate in the invisible interior of the organism," etc. We know that in the present day people are perfectly satisfied if they can find the name of the disease they are supposed to have, an idea cloaked in some wonderful technicality. An old Irishman walked into the clinic one day, and after giving his symptoms, said, "Doctor, what is the matter with me?" The physician answered, "Why, you have *Nux Vomica*," that being his remedy. Whereupon the old man said, "Well, I did think I had some wonderful disease or other." That is an outgrowth of the old-fashioned folly of naming sickness. Except in a few acute diseases no diagnosis can be made and no diagnosis need be made except that the patient is sick. The more one thinks of the name of a disease so-called the more one is beclouded in the search for a remedy, for then the mind is only upon the result of the disease, and not upon the image expressed in symptoms.

A patient of twenty-five years of age, with gravest inheritances, with twenty pages of symptoms, and with only symptoms to furnish an image of sickness, is perfectly curable if treated in time. After being treated there will be no pathological results; he will go on to old age without any tissue destruction. But that patient if not cured at that early age will take on disease results in accordance with the circumstances of his life and his inheritances. If he is a chimney sweep he will be subject to the disease peculiar to chimney sweeps. If she is a housemaid she will be subject to the disease peculiar to housemaids, etc. That patient has the same disease he had when he was born. This array of symptoms represents the same state before the pathological conditions have been formed as after. And it is true, if he has liver disease or brain disease or any of the many tissue changes that they call disease, you must go back and procure these very symptoms before you can make a prescription. Prescribing for the results of disease causes changes in the results of disease, but not in the sickness except to hurry its progress.

We will see peculiarities running through families. In the beginning is this primary state which is presented only by signs and symptoms, and the whole family needs the same remedy or a cognate of that remedy; but in one member of the family the condition runs to cancer, in another to phthisis, etc., but all from the same common foundation. This fundamental condition which underlies the diseases of the human race must be understood. Without a knowledge of this it will be impossible to understand the acute miasmatic diseases, which will be considered later.

It is a well-known fact that some persons are susceptible to one thing and some to another. If an epidemic comes upon the land only a few come down with it. Why are some protected and why do others take it? These things must be settled by the doctrines of Homœopathy. Idiosyncrasies must be accounted for. Many physicians waste their time searching after the things that make their patients sick. The sick man will be made sick under every circumstance, whereas the healthy man could live in a lazaretto. It is not the principal business of the physician to be hunting in the rivers and the cellars and examining the food we eat for the cause of disease. It is his duty to hunt out the symptoms of sickness until a remedy is found that covers the disorder. That remedy, which will produce on healthy man similar symptoms, is the master of the situation, is the necessary antidote, will overcome the sickness, restore the will and understanding to order and cure the patient.

To get at the real nature of the human economy, and to lead up from that to sickness, opens out a field for investigation in a most scientific way. Sickness can be learned by the study of the provings of drugs upon the healthy economy. Hahnemann made use of the information thus obtained when he stated that the mind is the key to the man. The symptoms of the mind have been found by all his followers to be the most important symptoms in a remedy and in a sickness. Man consists in what he thinks and what he loves and there is nothing else in man. If these two grand parts of man, the will and understanding, be separated it means insanity, disorder, death. All medicines operate upon the will and understanding first (sometimes extensively on both) affecting man in his ability to think or to will, and ultimately upon the tissues, the functions and sensations. In the study of *Aurum* we find the *affections* are most disturbed by that drug. Man's highest possible love is for his life. *Aurum* so destroys this that he does not love his life, he will commit suicide. *Argentum* on the other hand so destroys man's *understanding* that he is no longer rational; his memory is entirely ruined. So with every proved drug in the Materia Medica. We see them affecting first man's mind, and proceeding from the mind to the physical economy, to the outermost, to the skin, the hair, the nails. If medicines are not thus studied you will have no knowledge of them that you can carry with you. The Materia Medica has been established upon this basis.

Sickness must therefore be examined by a thorough scrutiny of the elements that make up morbid changes that exist in the likeness of drug symptoms. To the extent that drugs in provings upon healthy men have brought out symptoms on animal ultimates must we study sickness with the hope of adjusting remedies to sickness in man under the law of similars. Ultimate symptoms, function symptoms, sensorium symptoms and mind symptoms are all useful and none should be overlooked. The idea of sickness in man must be formed from the idea of sickness perceived in our Materia Medica. As we perceive the nature of sickness in a drug image, so must we perceive the nature of the sickness in a human being to be healed.

Therefore our idea of pathology must be adjusted to such a Materia Medica as we possess, and it must be discovered wherein these are similar in order to heal the sick. The totality of the symptoms written out carefully is all that we know of the internal nature of sickness. Then the proper administration of the similar remedy will constitute the art of healing.

LECTURE II

§ 2. The Highest Ideal of a Cure

The subject this morning relates to cure, to what the nature of a cure is. It is stated in the second paragraph of the *Organon* that

The highest ideal of a cure is rapid, gentle and permanent restoration of the health, or removal and annihilation of the disease in its whole extent, in the shortest, most reliable and most harmless way, on easily comprehensible principles.

If you were to ask a physician, who had not been trained in Homœopathy, of what a cure consists, his mind would only revolve around the idea of the disappearance of the pathological state; if an eruption on the skin were the given instance, the disappearance of the eruption from the skin under his treatment would be called a cure; if hemorrhoids, the removal of these would be called a cure; if constipation, the opening of the bowels would be called a cure; if some affection of the knee joint, an amputation above the knee would be considered a cure; or if it were an acute disease and the patient did not die, it would be considered a cure of the disease. And that is really the idea of the patient as it is derived from the physician. The patient will often wonder at the great skill of the physician in removing an eruption from the skin, and will go back again when the graver manifestations, the tissue changes threatening death, have come on as a consequence, and will say to the doctor: "You so wonderfully cured me of my skin disease, why cannot you cure of my liver trouble?" But this very scientific ignorant doctor has made a failure: he has driven what was upon the surface and harmless into the innermost precincts of the economy and the patient is going to die as a result of scientific ignorance.

There are three distinct points involved in this paragraph and these must be brought out. *Restoring health,* and not the removing of symptoms, is the first point. Restoring health has in view the establishment of order in a sick human being; removing symptoms has not in view a human being; removing the constipation, the hæmorrhoids, the white swelling of the knee, the skin disease or any local manifestation or particular sign of disease, or even the removal of a group of symptoms, does not have in view the restoration to health of the whole economy of man. If the removal of symptoms is not followed by a restoration to health, it cannot be called a cure. We learned in our last study that "the sole duty of the physician is to heal the sick," and therefore it is not his duty merely to remove the symptoms, to change the aspect of the symptoms, the appearance of the disease image, imagining that he has thereby established order. What a simple-minded creature he must be! What a groveller in muck and mire he must be, when he can meditate upon doing such things, even a moment! How different his actions would be if he but considered that every violent change which he produces in the aspect of the disease aggravates the interior nature of the disease, aggravates the sickness of the man and brings about an increase of suffering within him. The *patient* should be able to realize by his feelings and continue to say, that *he* is being restored to health, whenever a symptom is removed. There should be a corresponding inward improvement whenever an outward symptom has been caused to disappear, and this will be true whenever disease has been displaced by order.

The perfection of a cure consists, then, first in restoring health, and this is to be done *promptly, mildly* and *permanently*, which is the second point. The cure must be quick or speedy, it must be gentle, and it must be continuous or permanent. Whenever an outward symptom has been caused to disappear by violence, as by cathartics to remove constipation, it cannot be called mild or permanent, even if it is prompt. Whenever violent drugs are resorted to there is nothing mild in the action or the reaction that must follow. At the time this second paragraph of the *Organon* was written physicking was not so mild as at the present day; blood-letting, sweating, etc., were in vogue at the time Hahnemann wrote these lines. Medicine has changed somewhat in its appearance; physicians are now using sugar-coated pills and contriving to make medicines appear tasteless or tasteful; they are using concentrated alkaloids. But none of these things have been done because of the discovery of any principle; blood-letting and sweating were not abandoned on account of principle, for the old men deprecate their disuse, and often say they hope the time will come when they can again go back to the lancet. But the drugs of today are ten times more powerful than those formerly used, because more concentrated. The cocaine, sulphonal and numerous other modern concentrated products of the manufacturing chemists are extremely dangerous and their real action and reaction unknown. The chemical discoveries of petroleum have opened a field of destruction to human intelligence, to the understanding and to the will, because these products are slowly and insidiously violent. When drugs were used that were instantly dangerous and violent the action was manifest, it showed upon the surface, and the common people saw it. But the patient of the present day goes through more dangerous drugging, because it destroys the mind. The apparent benefits produced by these drugs are never permanent. They may in some cases seem to be permanent, but then it is because upon the economy has been engrafted a new and most insidious disease, more subtle and more tenacious than the manifestation that was upon the externals and it is because of this tenacity that the original symptoms remain away. The disease in its nature, its *esse*, has not been changed; it is still there, causing the internal destruction of the man, but its manifestation has been changed, and there has been added to this natural disease a drug disease, more serious than the former.

The manner of cure can only be mild if it flows in the stream of natural direction, establishing order and thereby removing disease. The direction of old-fashioned medicine is like pulling a cat up a hill by the tail; whereas, the treatment that is mild, gentle and permanent, flows with the stream, scarcely producing a ripple; it adjusts the internal disorder and the outermost of man returns to order. Everything becomes orderly from the interior. The curative medicine does not act violently upon the economy, but establishes its action in a mild manner; but while the action is mild and gentle, very often that which follows, which is the reaction, is a turmoil, especially when the work of traditional medicine is being undone and former states are being re-established.

The third point is "upon *principles* that are at once plain and intelligible." This means law, it means fixed principles; it means a law as certain as that of gravitation; not guess work, empiricism, or roundabout methods, or a cut-and-dried use of drugs as laid down by the last manufacturer. Our principles have never changed, they have always been the same and will remain the same. To become acquainted with these principles and doctrines, with fixed knowledges, with exactitude or method, to become acquainted with medicines that never change their properties, and to become acquainted with their action, is the all-important aim in homœopathic study. When one has learned these principles, and continues to practice them, they grow brighter and stronger. The use of these fixed principles is the removal of disease, the restoration to health in a mild, prompt and permanent manner.

If one were to ask an allopathic graduate in this class how he could demonstrate that he had cured somebody, the answer could only be such as I have mentioned already, viz., that the patient did not die, or that the manifestations prescribed for had disappeared. If one were to ask a physician trained in homœopathic principles the same question, one would find that there are means of distinctly demonstrating why he knows his patient is better. You would naturally expect, if it is the interior of man that is disordered in sickness, and not his tissues primarily, that the interior must first be turned into order and the exterior last. The first of man is his voluntary and the second of man is his understanding, the last of man is his outermost; from his centre to his circumference, to his organs, his skin, hair, nails, etc. This being true, the cure must proceed from centre to circumference. From centre to circumference is *from above downward,* from *within outwards,* from more important to less important organs, from the head to the hands and feet. Every homœopathic practitioner who understands the art of healing, knows that symptoms which go off in these directions remain away permanently. Moreover, he knows that symptoms which *disappear in the reverse order of their coming* are removed permanently. It is thus he knows that the patient did not merely get well in spite of the treament, but that he was cured by the action of the remedy. If a homœopathic physician goes to the bedside of a patient and, upon observing the onset of the symptoms and the course of the disease, sees that the symptoms do not follow this order after his remedy, he knows that he has had but little to do with the course of things.

But if, on the contrary, he observes after the administration of his medicine that the symptoms take a reverse course, then he knows that his medicine has had to do with it, because if the disease were allowed to run its course such a result would not take place. The progression of chronic diseases is from the surface to the centre. All chronic diseases have their first manifestations upon the surface, and from that to the innermost of man. Now in the proportion in which they are thrown back upon the surface it is to be seen that the patient is recovering. Here it is that the turmoil

spoken of above follows the true homœopathic remedy, and the
ignorant do not desire their old outward symptom to be brought
back even when it is known as the only possible form of cure.
Complaints of the heart and chest and head must in recovery be
accompanied by manifestations upon the surface, in the extremities, upon the skin, nails and hair. Hence you will find that these
parts become diseased when patients are getting well; the hair falls
out or eruptions come upon the skin. In cases of rheumatism of the
heart you find, if the patient is recovering, that his knees become
rheumatic, and he may say: "Doctor, I could walk all over the
house when you first came to me, but now I cannot walk, my
joints are so swollen." If the doctor does not know that that means
recovery he will make a prescription that will drive the rheumatism
away from the feet and knees and it will go back to the heart and
the patient will die; and it need hardly be stated that the traditional doctor does not know this, as he resorts to this plan as his
regular and only plan of treatment, and in the most innocent way
kills the patient. This is a simple illustration of how it is possible
for the interiors of man to cease to be affected and the exteriors to
become affected. It may be impossible for the man to be entirely
cured, it may be impossible for this state to pass off, but that is the
direction of its passing off and there is no other course. If the
patient is incurable, while the means used are mild he may experience great suffering in the evolution of his disease, in the course
of his partial recovery. To him it may not appear mild, but the
means that were used were mild. In acute diseases we do not observe so much distress after prescribing as we see in old incurable
cases, in deep-seated chronic complaints that have existed a long
time. The return of the outward manifestations upon the extremities are noticed in such cases where they have been suppressed. To
illustrate: there are many patients who have had rheumatism in
the hands and feet, in the wrists and knees and elbows, who have
been rubbed and stimulated with lotions and strong liniments, with
chloroform, with evaporating lotions, with cooling applications,
until the rheumatism of the extremities has disappeared to a great
extent, but every physician knows that as the disappearance of his
rheumatism progresses cardiac symptoms are likely to occur. When
this patient is prescribed for the rheumatism of the extremities
must come back or the heart will not be relieved. That is true of
every condition that has been upon the extremities and driven in

by local treatment. Just as surely as you live and observe the action of homœopathic remedies upon man, so surely will you see these symptoms come back. The patient will return and say: "Doctor, I have the same symptoms that I had when I was treated by Dr. So-and-so for rheumatism." This comes out in practice nearly every day.

It requires a little explanation to the patient, and if he is intelligent enough to understand it, he will wait for the remedy to act. But the physician who thinks most of his pocketbook will say: "If I don't give him a liniment to put on that limb he will go off and get another physician." Now let me tell you right here is the beginning of evil. You had better trust to the intelligence of humanity and trust that he will stay and be cured. If you have learned to prescribe for the patient even though he suffer, if you have learned what is right and do not do it, it is a violation of conscience.

This paragraph appeals to man's integrity; it is said in the last line "on principles that are at once plain and intelligible." Just as soon as you leave out integrity, and believe that a man can do just as he pleases, you leave out everything that pertains to principle and you leave out the foundation of success. But when these principles are carried out, when a man has made himself thoroughly conversant with the Materia Medica and thoroughly intelligent in its application, when he is circumspect in his very interior life as to the carrying out of these principles, then he will lead himself into a use that is most delightful, because by such means he may cause diseases to disappear, and may win the lasting friendship and respect of a class of people worth working for. He has more than that, he has a clear conscience with all that belongs to it; he is living a life of innocence. When he lives such a life he does not allow himself to wink at the notions that are carried out in families, as, for example, how to prevent the production of offspring, how to avoid bearing children, how to separate man and wife by teaching them the nasty little methods of avoiding the bringing forth of offspring. The meddling with these vices and the advocating of them will prevent the father and mother from being cured of their chronic diseases. Unless people lead an orderly life they will not be cured of their chronic diseases. It is your duty as physicians to inculcate such principles among them that they may live an orderly life. The physician who does not know what order is ought not to be trusted.

It is the duty of the physician, then, first to find out what is in man that is disorder, and then to restore him to health; and this return to health, which is a perfect cure, is to be accomplished by means that are mild, that are orderly, that flow gently like the life force itself, turning the internal of man into order, with fixed principles as his guide, and by the homœopathic remedy.

LECTURE III

§ 3. Perfection of what is Curable in Disease, Curative in Medicine and the Application of Last to First

Organon Sec. 3. If the physician clearly perceives what is to be cured in diseases, that is to say, in every individual case of disease: if he clearly perceives what is curative in medicines, that is to say, in each individual medicine; and if he knows how to adapt, according to clearly-defined principles, what is curative in medicines to what he has discovered to be undoubtedly morbid in the patient, so that recovery must ensure—to adapt it as well in respect to the suitability of the medicine most appropriate according to its mode of action to the case before him, as also in respect to the exact mode of preparation and quantity of it required, and the proper period for repeating the dose; if, finally, he knows the obstacles to recovery in each case and is aware how to remove them so that the restoration may be permanent: *then he understands how to treat judiciously and rationally, and he is a true practitioner of the healing art.*

The translator has correctly used here the word "perceive," which is to see into, not merely to look upon with the external eye, but to clearly understand, to apprehend with the mind and understanding. If Hahnemann had said "see" instead of "perceive," it might have been taken to mean seeing with the eye a tumor to be cut or, by opening the abdomen, to see the diseased kidney, or, by examination of the urine, to see that there is albumen or sugar present, by removing which in some mysterious way the patient would be cured. It is evident by this that Hahnemann did not look upon pathological change or morbid anatomy as that which in disease constitutes the curative indication. The physician must perceive in the disease that which is to be cured, and the curative indication in each particular case of disease is *the totality of the symptoms*, *i.e.*, the disease is represented or expressed by the totality of the symptoms, and this totality (which is the speech of nature) is not itself the *esse* of the disease, it only represents the disorder in the internal economy. This totality, which is really external, a manifestation in the tissues, will arrange itself into form to present, as it were, to the physician the internal disorder.

The first thing to be considered in a case is, What are the curative indications in this case? What signs and symptoms call the physician's attention as curative signs and symptoms? This means not every manifestation is a curative indication. The results of disease occurring in the tissues, in chronic diseases, such as cancerous changes, tumors, etc., are of such a character that they cannot constitute curative signs; but those things which are curable, which are capable of change, which can be materially affected by the administration of remedies, the physician must know; they are the curative indications.

The physician ought to have a well-grounded idea of government and law to which there are no exceptions; he ought to see the cause of disease action to be from centre to circumference, from the innermost of the man to his outermost. If law and government are present, then law directs every act taking place in the human system. Every government is from the centre to the circumference. Look at it politically. Whenever the system of central political government is not bowed to, anarchy and loss of confidence prevail. There are also commercial centres. We must recognize London, Paris, and New York as centres of commercial government in their different spheres. Even the spider entrenches himself in his web and governs his universe from the centre. There cannot be two governments; such would lead to confusion. There is but one unit in every standard. In man the centre of government is in the cerebrum and from it every nerve cell is governed. From it all actions take place for good or evil, for order or disorder; from it disease begins and from it begins the healing process. It is not from external things that man becomes sick, not from bacteria nor environment, but from causes in himself. If the homœopath does not see this, he cannot have a true perception of disease. Disorder in the vital economy is the primary state of affairs, and this disorder manifests itself by signs and symptoms.

In perceiving what is to be cured in disease one must proceed from generals to particulars, study disease in its most general features, not as seen upon one particular individual, but upon the whole human race. We will endeavour to bring this idea before the mind by taking as an example one of the acute miasms, not for the purpose of diagnosis, as this is easy, but to arrange it for a therapeutic examination. Let us take an epidemic, say, of scarlet fever, or grippe, or measles, or cholera. If the epidemic is entirely different from anything that has hitherto appeared in the neighbourhood it is at first confusing. From the first few cases the physician has a very vague idea of this disease, for he sees only a fragment of it, and gets only a portion of its symptoms. But the epidemic spreads and many patients are visited, and twenty individuals have perhaps been closely observed. Now if the physician will write down all the symptoms that have been present in each case in a schematic form, arranging the mind symptoms of the different patients under "mind" and the head symptoms under "head," and so on, following Hahnemann's method, they—considered collectively—will present one image, as if one man had expressed all the symptoms, and in this way he will have that particular disease in schematic form. If he places opposite each symptom a number corresponding to the number of patients in which that symptom occurred, he will find out the essential features of the epidemic. For example, twenty patients had aching in the bones, and at once he sees that that symptom is a part of this epidemic. All the patients had catarrhal affections of the eye, and a measly rash, and these also must be recorded as pathognomonic symptoms. And so by taking the entire scheme and studying it as a whole, as if one patient had experienced all the symptoms, he is able to perceive how this new disease, this contagious disease, affects the human race, and each particular patient, and he is able to predicate of it what is general and what is particular. Every new patient has a few new symptoms; he has put his own stamp on that disease. Those symptoms that run through all are the pathognomonic symptoms; those which are rare are the peculiarities of the different people. This totality represents to the human mind, as nearly as possible, the nature of this sickness, and it is this nature that the therapeutist must have in mind.

Now let him take the next step, which is to find in general the remedies that correspond to this epidemic. By the aid of a repertory he will write after each one of these symptoms all the remedies that have produced that symptom. Having in this way gone through the entire schema, he can then begin to eliminate for practical purposes, and he will see that six or seven remedies run through the picture, and, therefore, are related to the epidemic, corresponding to its whole nature. This may be called the group of epidemic remedies for that particular epidemic, and with these he will manage to cure nearly all his cases. The question now arises, which one is the remedy for each individual case? When he has worked out the half dozen remedies he can go through the Materia Medica and get their individual pictures so fixed in his

head that he can use them successfully. Thus he proceeds from
generals to particulars, and there is no other way to proceed in
homœopathy. He is called to a family with half a dozen patients
in bed from this epidemic, and he finds a little difference in each
case so that one remedy is indicated in one patient and another
remedy in another patient. There is no such thing in homœopathy
as administering one of these remedies to all in the family because
of a diagnostic name. Now, while one of the remedies in the epidemic group will most likely be indicated in many cases, yet if
none of these should fit the patient, the physician must return to
his original anamnesis to see which one of the other remedies is
suitable. Very rarely will a patient demand a remedy not in the
anamnesis. Every remedy has in itself a certain state of peculiarities that identifies it as an individual remedy, and the patient has
also a certain state of peculiarities that identifies him as an individual patient, and so the remedy is fitted to the patient. No remedy
must be given because it is in the list, for the list has only been
made as a means of facilitating the study of that epidemic. Things
can only be made easy by an immense amount of hard work, and
if you do the drudgery in the beginning of an epidemic, the prescribing for your cases will be rapid, and you will find your
remedies abort cases of sickness, make malignant cases simple, so
simplify scarlet fever that classification would be impossible, stop
the course of typhoids in a week, and cure remittent fevers in a
day.

If the physician does not work this scheme out on paper he must
do it in the mind, but if he becomes very busy and sees a large
number of cases it will be too much to carry in the mind. You will
be astonished to find that if you put an epidemic on paper you will
forever be able to carry the knowledge of it in mind. I have done
this, and have been surprised to find that after a dozen references
to it I did not need it any more.

Now you may say, how is this in regard to typhoid fever? It is
not a new disease, it is an old form. The old practitioner has
unconsciously made an anamnesis of his typhoid cases, he has
unconsciously written it out in his mind and carries it around. It is
not difficult to work out the group of typhoid remedies, and from
this group he works. The same is true with regard to measles, certain remedies correspond to the nature of measles, i.e., when
studied by its symptoms and not by name.

Of course, every now and then will come up a rare and singular case, which will compel you to go outside of the usual group. Never allow yourself to be so cramped that you cannot go outside of the medicines that you have settled upon as medicines, say, for measles. All your nondescript cases of course will get *Pulsatilla*, because it is so similar to the nature of measles, but it does not do to be too limited or routine, but be sure in administering a remedy that the indications are clear. Every busy practitioner thinks of *Ailanthus, Apis, Belladonna* and *Sulphur* for malignant cases of scarlet fever, and yet he has often to go outside of that group.

So the physician perceives in the disease what it is that constitutes the curative indication.

This presents itself to his mind only when he is clearly conversant with the nature of the sickness, as, for instance, with the nature of scarlet fever, of measles, of typhoid fever,—the zymosis, the blood changes, etc., so that when they arrive he is not surprised; when the typhoid state progresses he expects the tympanitic abdomen, the diarrhœa, the continued fever, the rash, the delirium and unconsciousness. These things stand out as the nature of typhoid. When, therefore, he goes to the Materia Medica he at once calls up before his mind this nature of typhoid, and so is able to pick out the remedies that have such a nature. He sees in *Phosphorus, Rhus, Bryonia, Baptisia, Arsenicum,* etc., low forms of fever, corresponding to the typhoid condition. But when the patient jumps away out of the ordinary group of remedies, then it is that he has to go outside of the beaten track and find another remedy that also corresponds to the nature of typhoid fever.

By these remarks I am endeavouring to hold up before you what the physician regards as the curative indications of disease. First he sees the disease in general as to its nature, and then when an individual has this disease this individual will present in his own peculiarities the peculiar features of that disease. The homœopath is in the habit of studying the slightest shades of difference between patients, the little things that point to the remedy. If we looked upon disease only as the old-school physician sees it we would have no means of distinction, but it is because of the little peculiarities manifested by every individual patient, through his inner life, through everything he thinks, that the homœopath is enabled to individualize.

"If the physician clearly perceives what is curative in medicines, that is to say, in each individual medicine." Here again he progresses from general to particulars. He cannot become acquainted clearly with the action of medicines individually until he becomes acquainted with the action of medicines collectively, proceeding from a collective study to a particular. This is to be done by studying provings. Suppose we were to start out in this class and make a proving of some unknown drug. It would be expected that you would all bring out the same symptoms, but the same general features would run through this class of provers; each individual would have his own peculiarities. No. 1 might bring out the symptoms of the mind more clearly than No. 2; No. 2 might bring out the symptoms of the bowels more clearly than No. 1; No. 3 might bring out heal symptoms very strongly, etc. Now if these were collected together as if one man had proved the medicine, we would then have an image of that medicine. If we had a hundred provers we would go through the whole nature of this remedy and perceive how it affected the human race, how it acted as a unit.

What I have said before about studying the nature of disease must be applied to the study of the nature of a remedy.

A remedy is in condition to be studied as a whole when it is on paper, the mind symptoms under one head, the symptoms of the scalp under another, and so on throughout the entire body in accordance with Hahnemann's schema. We may go on adding to it, developing it, noting which of the symptoms or groups of symptoms are the most prominent. A remedy is not fully proved until it has permeated and made sick all regions of the body. When it has done this it is ready for study and for use. Many of our provings are only fragments and are given in the books for what they are worth. Hahnemann followed up in full all the remedies that he handed down to us; in these the symptoms have been brought out upon the entire man. Each individual medicine must be studied in that way, as to how it changes the human race.

To understand the nature of the chronic miasms, psora, syphilis and sycosis, the homœopath must proceed in identically the same way as with the acute. Hahnemann has put on paper an image of psora. For eleven years he collected the symptoms of those patients who were undoubtedly psoric and arranged them in schematic form until the nature of this great miasm became apparent. Following upon that he published antipsoric remedies which in their nature have a similarity to psora. To be a really successful physician the homœopath must proceed along the same lines in regard to syphilis and sycosis.

Now, when the physician sees, as it were, in an image, the nature of disease, when he is acquainted with every disease to which we are subject, and when he sees the nature of the remedies in common use, just as clearly as he perceives disease, then on listening to the symptoms of a sick man he knows instantly the remedies that have produced upon healthy man symptoms similar to these. This is what paragraph 3 teaches; it looks towards making the homœopathic physician so intelligent that when he goes to the bedside of a patient he can clearly perceive the nature of disease and the nature of the remedy. It is a matter of perception; he sees with his understanding. When a physician understands the nature of disease and of remedies, then it is that he will be skilful.

is no inward flow. Man is protected against things flowing in from the outward toward the centre. All disease flows from the innermost to the outermost, and unless drug substances are prepared in a form to do this they can neither produce nor cure disease. There are miasms in the universe, acute and chronic. The chronic, which have no tendency toward recovery, are three, psora, syphilis and sycosis; we shall study these later. Outside of acute and chronic miasms there are only the results of disease to be considered. The miasms are contagious; they flow from the innermost to the outermost; and while they exist in organs yet they are imperceptible, for they cannot exist in man unless they exist in form subtle enough to operate upon the innermost of man's physical nature. The correspondence of this innermost cannot be discovered by man's eye, by his fingers, or by any of his senses, neither can any disease cause be found with the microscope. Disease can only be perceived by its results, and it flows from within out, from centre to circumference, from the seat of government to the outermost. Hence cure must be from within out.

In our civil government we see the likeness to this. Let any great disturbance come upon our government at Washington and see how, like lightning, this is felt to the circumference of the nation. How the whole country becomes shaken and disturbed as if by disease if it is an evil government. If the government be good, we observe it in the form of improvement, and everybody is benefited by it. If in the great centres of commerce, London, Paris or New York, some great crash or crisis takes place, how the very circumference that depends upon these centres is shaken, as it were, by disease. Every little political office depends upon Washington, and that order must be preserved most thoroughly. The sheriff and constable, the judge and the court, are little governments dependent upon the law that is formed by the state. The law of the state would be nothing if the centre of our government at Washington were dethroned by another nation. All the law and principles in Pennsylvania depended upon the permanency and orderliness of the government in Washington, and there is a series from Washington to Harrisburg and from Harrisburg to Philadelphia. There can be no broken link.

It is now seen what is to be understood by order and directions, and that there are directions; nothing can flow in from the outermost to affect the innermost. Disturb one of the courts in Philadelphia and this does not disturb the country or the constitutional government. If the finger is burnt this does not to any great extent disturb the constitutional government of the man, but the constitutional government repairs it. It is not a disease, it does not rack the whole frame. It is only that which shakes the whole economy, disturbs the government, which is a disease. So man may have his hand cut off without the system being disturbed, but let a little disease, measles for example, flow in from the centre and his whole economy is racked. Old-fashioned medicine talks of experience, but is entirely dependent on the eyes and fingers; appearances are wonderfully deceptive. If you examine any acute miasm you may know what it looks like, but the *esse* of it cannot be discovered by any of the senses.

We have seen that everything is governed from the centre. Now what comes in the direction of law, what comes from principle, comes from the centre, is flowing in accordance with order and can be confirmed by experience. To apply it more practically, what we learn from the use of the law of homœopathics, what we observe after learning that law and the doctrines that relate to it— all our subsequent experience, confirms the principles. For example, every experience with *Bryonia* makes *Bryonia* so much brighter in mind. With experience one grows stronger; one does not change or alter with every mood, but becomes firmly established. If everything tends to disturb the mind, that means that you are in a state of folly or that you are insane; it may be a little of both. A man that relies on experience to guide him never knows; his mind is constantly changing, never settled; it has no validity. Validity is something absolutely essential to science. It is necessary for homœopaths to look upon law as valid and not upon man, as there is no man valid. In Homœopathy it is the very principle itself that is valid, and things that are not in accordance with principle should not be admitted.

We see from all this the necessity of potentization. All causes are so refined in character, so subtle in their nature, that they can operate from centre to circumference, operate upon man's interiors and from the interior to the very exterior. The coarser things cannot permeate the skin. Man's skin is an envelope, protecting him against contagion from coarser materials; but against the immaterial substance he is protected only when in perfect health. In an unguarded moment he suffers, and this is the nature and quality of disease cause. It can only flow into man from the centre and towards the outermost in a way to disturb his government. The disturbance of government is a disturbance of order, and this is all there is of sickness, and we have only to follow this out to find that the very house man lives in, and his cells, are becoming deranged. Changes are the result of disorder and end in breaking down, degeneration, etc.; pus cells and the various forms of degeneration are only the result of disorder. So long as order and harmony go on perfectly, so long the tissues are in a state of health, the metamorphosis is healthy, the tissue change is normal, the physiological state is maintained.

We can only comprehend the nature of disease, and tissue changes the result of disease, by going back to its beginning. The study of etiology in the old school is a wonderful farce, because it begins with nothing. It is an assumption that tissue changes are the disease. From the doctrines of Homœopathy it will be seen that morbid anatomy, no matter where it occurs, must be considered to be the result of disease.

All curable diseases make themselves known to the physician by signs and symptoms. When the disease does not make itself known in signs and symptoms, and its progress is in the interior, we at once perceive that that man is in a very precarious condition. Conditions of the body that are incurable are such very often as have no external signs or symptoms.

In the fourth paragraph Hahnemann says: "The physician is likewise a preserver of health if he knows the things that derange health and cause disease and how to remove them from persons in health." If the physician believes that causes are external, if he believes that the material changes in the body are the things that disturb health, are the fundamental cause of sickness, he will undertake to remove these, e.g., he will cut off hemorrhoids or remove the tumor. But these are not objects Hahnemann means. The objects he means are invisible and can only be known by signs and symptoms. Of course, it is quite right for the physician to remove those things that are external to the sick man and are troubling him. These are not disease, but they are in a measure disturbing him and making him sick, aggravating his chronic miasm so that it will progress and destroy. These are outward obstacles and not the disease, but in this way man is very often rendered more susceptible to acute miasms. The things "which keep up disease" relate more particularly to external things. There are conditions in man's life which keep up or encourage man's disorder. The disorder is from the interior, but many of the disturbances that aggravate the disorders are external. The cause of disorder is internal, and is of such quality that it affects the government from the interior, while the coarser things are such as can disturb more especially the body, such as improperly selected food, living in damp houses, etc. It is hardly worth while to dwell upon these things, because any ordinary physician is sufficiently well versed in hygiene to remove from his patients the external obstacles.

In the fifth paragraph Hahnemann says: "Useful to the physician in assisting him to cure are the particulars of the most probable *exciting cause* of the acute disease, etc." The probable exciting cause is the inflowing of the cause as an invisible, immaterial substance, which, having fastened upon the interior, flows from the very centre to the outermost of the economy, creating additional disorder. These miasms all require a given time to operate before they can affect the external man, and this time is called the prodromal stage.

This is true of psora, syphilis and sycosis and of every acute contagious disease known to man. While the influx is upon the innermost of the physical man it is not apparent, but when it begins to operate upon his nerves and tissues, affecting him in his outermost, then it becomes apparent. Each miasm produces upon the human economy its own characteristics, just as every drug produces upon the human economy its own characteristics. Hahnemann says that these must be recognized, that the homœopathic physician must be familiar enough with disease cause, with disease manifestations and drug manifestations to be able to remove them in accordance with principles fixed and certain. There should be no hypothesis nor opinion, neither should simple experience have a place.

If the physician is dealing with acute cases he must take into consideration the nature of the case as a malady, and so also with chronic cases. It is supposed that he is conversant with the disease from having observed the symptoms of a great many cases, and is therefore able to hold before the mind the image of the disease. When he is thoroughly conversant with the very image of the sicknesses that exist upon the human race he is then prepared to study Materia Medica. All the imitations of miasms are found in drugs.

There is no miasm of the human race that does not have its imitation in drugs. The animal kingdom has in itself the image of sickness, and the vegetable and mineral kingdoms in like manner, and if man were perfectly conversant with the substances of these three kingdoms he could treat the whole human race.

By application the physician must fill his mind with images that correspond to the sicknesses of the human race. It is being conversant with symptomatology, with the symptom images of disease, that makes one a physician. The books of the present time are defective, in that they ignore symptomatology and do not furnish us an image of the sickness. They are extensively treatises on pathology, upon heredity, with very little of the patient himself. If we go back to earlier times, when the physician did not know so much about the microscope, when he did not examine into the cause of disease so minutely, we will find in such works as "*Watson's Practice*" much better descriptions of sickness. Watson stands at the bedside and relates what his patients look like, and hence it is a grand old book for the homœopathic physician. Chambers, in his lectures at St. Mary's Hospital, London, also relates with accuracy the appearance of the patient. At the present time the old-school physician says: "I want to know nothing about your symptoms; take this and go to the first drug store and have it filled." This is the state of things at the present time, a look at the tongue, a feel of the pulse, and "take this," handing a prescription to be filled at the nearest pharmacy. Is that observing the sick? Can such a man be the guardian of the sick, when it requires time to bring out every little detail of sickness, and a nervous girl is driven off and never permitted to tell her symptoms? Such patients have told me after an hour's conversation and taking of symptoms: "The other doctor told me I had hysteria, that there was nothing the matter with me, that I was just nervous." That is what modern pathology leads men to think and say. Everything is denied that cannot be discovered by the senses; hence this false science has crept upon us until it is a typical folly. As to the end of sickness, what sickness will do is of no great matter, because by the symptoms we have perceived the nature of the illness and may safely trust to the remedy. If no remedy be applied to check the progress of the disease it may localize in the heart, lungs or kidneys, but the *nature* of the sickness exists in that state of disordered government expressed by signs and symptoms.

LECTURE V

§ 5. Discrimination as to Maintaining External Causes and Surgical Cases

We wish to revert for a short time to the fourth paragraph, in which Hahnemann says: "The physician is likewise a preserver of health if he knows the things that derange health and cause disease, and how to remove them from persons in health."

The Homœopathic physician is a failure if he does not discriminate. It seems that among the earliest things he must learn is to "Render unto Cæsar the things that are Cæsar's," to keep everything in its place, to keep everything in order. This little paragraph might seem to relate to nothing but hygiene. One of the most superficial things in it is to say that persons about to be made sick from bad habits should break off their bad habits, they should move from damp houses, they should plug their sewers or have traps put in if they are being poisoned with sewer gas. It is everybody's duty to do these things, but especially the physician's, and we might almost let it go with the saying. To prevent coffee drinking, vinegar drinking, etc. is a superficial thing; but in this way he may preserve health.

To discriminate, then, is a most important thing. To illustrate it in a general way we might say that one who is suffering from conscience does not need a surgeon. You might say he needs a priest. One who is sick in his vital force needs a physician. He who has a lacerated wound, or a broken bone, or deformities, has need of a surgeon. If his tooth must come out he must have a surgeon dentist. What would be thought of a man who, on being sent for a surgeon to set an injured man's bones should go for a carpenter to mend the roof of the man's house? If the man's house alone needs mending then he needs a carpenter and not a surgeon. The physician must discriminate between the man and his house, and between the repair of man and the repair of his house. It is folly to give medicine for a lacerated wound, to attempt to close up a deep wound with a dose of remedy. Injuries from knives, hooks, etc., affect the house the man lives in and must be attended to by the surgeon. When the gross exterior conditions which are brought on from exterior causes complicated with the interior man then medicine is required. If the physician acts also as a surgeon he must know when he is to perform his functions as a surgeon, and when he must keep back as a surgeon. He should sew up a wound, but should not burn out an ulcer with Nitrate of Silver. If he is not able to discriminate, and on every ulcer he plasters his external applications, he is not a preserver of health. When signs and symptoms are present the physician is needed, because these come from the interior to the exterior. But if his condition is brought on only from external causes, the physician must delay action and let the surgeon do his work. Yet we see around us that physicians bombard the house the man lives in and have no idea of treating the man. They are no more than carpenters, they attempt to repair the roof, put on boards and bandages, and yet by their bandaging the man from head to foot they often do an improper thing.

The physician must know the things that derange health and remove them. If a fang of an old tooth causes headache day and night that cause must be removed. To prescribe when a splinter is pressing on a nerve and leave the splinter in would be foolishness and criminal negligence. The aim should be to discriminate and remove external causes and turn into order internal causes. A man comes for treatment, and he is living on deviled crabs and lobster salad and other trash too rich for the stomach of a dog. If we keep on giving Nux Vomica to that man we are foolish. If a man who has been living viciously stops it he can be helped, but so long as that external cause is not removed the physician is not using discrimination. Vicious habits, bad living, living in damp houses are externals and must be removed. When a man avoids these externals, is cleanly, carefully chooses his food, has a comfortable home, and is still miserable, he must be treated from within.

You know how we are maligned and lied about. You have heard it said about some strict homœopath, "He tried to set a broken leg with the c.m. potency of Mercury. What a poor fool!" But still outside of such an instance this discrimination is an important matter. You must remember it especially when busy, as at times it will be hard to decide. This kind of diagnosis is important, because it settles between things external and internal. Every physician does not discriminate thus, for if he did there would not be so many poultices and murderous external applications used. Among those who do not discriminate are those who apply medicines externally and give them internally.

Now we return to the fifth paragraph, which reads:

Useful to the physician in assisting him to cure are the particulars of the most probable *exciting cause* of the acute disease, as also the most significant points in the whole history of the chronic disease to enable him to discover its *fundamental cause*, which is generally due to a chronic miasm. In these investigations the ascertainable physical constitution of the patient (especially when the disease is chronic), his moral and intellectual character, his occupation, mode of living and habits, his social and domestic relations, his age, sexual functions, etc., are to be taken into consideration.

Little is known of the real exciting causes. Acute affections are divided into two classes (1) those that are miasmatic, which are true diseases, and (2) those that may be called mimicking sickness. The living in damp houses, grief, bad clothing, etc.; and the causes being latter have no definite cause, are produced by external causes such as removed the patient recovers. But the first, the acute miasms have a distinct course to run. They have a *prodromal* period, a period of *progress* and a period of decline, if not so severe as to cause the patient's death. Measles, scarlet fever, whooping cough, smallpox, etc., are examples of acute miasms. The physician must also be acquainted with the chronic miasms, psora, syphilis and sycosis, which we will study later. These have like the acute, a prodromal period and a period of progress, but unlike the acute they have no period of decline. When the times and circumstances are favourable the chronic miasm becomes quiescent, but adverse times rouse it into activity, and each time it is aroused the condition is worse than it was at the previous exacerbation. In this paragraph Hahnemann teaches that the chronic miasms are the fundamental cause of the acute miasms, which is to say, if there were no chronic miasms there would be no acute. It is in the very nature of a chronic miasm to predispose man to acute diseases, and the acute diseases are as fuel added to an unquenchable fire. Acute diseases then exist from specific causes co-operating with susceptibility. We do not recognize measles or scarlet fever except in sick people. Their influence might exist in the atmosphere, but we cannot see it. So apart from the subjects that take and develop them we could not know that there were such diseases. If there were no children on the earth susceptible to measles we would have no measles, and if there were no chronic miasms there would be no susceptibility. We will take up the subject of susceptibility later.

Psora is the cause of all contagion. If man had not had psora he would not have had the other two chronic miasms, but psora, the oldest, became the basis of the others. The physicians of the present day do not comprehend Hahnemann's definition of psora, they think it meant an itch vesicle or some sort of tetter. They regard itch as only the result of the action of a bug that crawls in the skin making vesicles, all of which is external. This is quite in keeping with man's present form of investigation, because he can comprehend only that which he discovers by his senses. Hahnemann's idea of psora, as we shall see when we come to study it, is wholly different from these perverted views. Psora corresponds to that state of man in which he has so disordered his economy to the very uttermost that he has become susceptible to every surrounding influence. The other day I used the illustration of civil government, and said if our civil government is evil in its centre it will be in disorder in its uttermost. So if a man is evil in his very interiors, *i.e.*, in his will and understanding, and the result of this evil flows into his life, he is in a state of disorder. Let man exist for thousands of years thinking false theories and bringing them into his life, and his life will become one of disorder.

Later we will be able to show that this disordered condition of the economy is the underlying and fundamental state of the nature of psora which ultimates upon the body in tissue changes. Suppose a man starts out and believes that it is right for him to live upon a certain kind of food that is very distasteful to him; he lives upon that diet until he thinks (from his belief) that he really loves it, and in time his very outermost becomes as morbid as he is himself. When man is insane in his interior it is only a question of time and his body will take on the results of insanity because the interior of man forms the exterior. If the interior is insane the exterior is distorted, and is only suitable to the kind of insane or disordered life that dwells in it. False in the interior, false in the exterior, so that the body becomes, as it were, false. This is speaking from analogy, but you will come to see that it is actually true.

Each and everything that appears before the eyes is but the representative of its cause, and there is no cause except in the interior. Cause does not flow from the outermost of man to the interior, because man is protected against such a state of affairs. Causes exist in such subtle form that they cannot be seen by the eye. There is no disease that exists of which the cause is known to man by the eye or by the microscope. Causes are infinitely too fine to be observed by any instrument of precision. They are so immaterial that they correspond to and operate upon the interior nature of man, and they are ultimated in the body in the form of tissue changes that are recognized by the eye. Such tissue changes must be understood as the results of disease only or the physician will never perceive what disease cause is, what disease is, what potentization is, or what the nature of life is. This is what Hahnemann meant when he speaks of the fundamental causes as existing in chronic miasms.

Just as soon as man lives a disorderly life he is susceptible to outside influences, and the¹ more disorderly he lives the more susceptible he becomes to the atmosphere he lives in. When man thinks in a disorderly way he carries out his life in a disorderly way, and makes himself sick by disorderly habits of thinking and living. This deranged mental state Hahnemann most certainly recognizes, for he tells us everywhere in his teaching to pay most attention to the mental state. We must begin with such signs as represent to the mind the beginning of sickness, and this beginning will be found in the mental disorder as represented by signs and symptoms, and as it flows on we have the coarser manifestations of disease. The more that disease ultimates itself in the outward form the coarser it is and the less it points the physician to the remedy. The more mental it is the more signs there are to direct the physician to the remedy.

"In these investigations the ascertainable physical constitution of the patient, etc., are to be taken into consideration." This is the second state following the first one disordered. This deals with the outermost, it relates to externals. You have to consider both the internal and external man; that is, you have to consider causes that operate in this disordered innermost, and then the ultimates which constitute the outward appearance, particularly when the affection is chronic. These two things must be considered, the nature or *esse* of the disease and its appearance. At the present day diseases are named in the books from their appearance and not from any idea as to what the nature or *esse* of sickness is, hence the disease names in our books are misleading, as they do not have reference to the sick man but to ultimates. If the disease has terminated in the liver, numerous names are applied to the liver; if in the kidney or heart, these organs have names applied to them, and such terminations are called diseases. Consumption is a tubercular state of the lungs, which is but the result of an internal disorder which was operating in the interior long before the breakdown of tissue.

The physicians of these days will tell you that they go back to the cause, but they present no cause; they only bring up the superficial conditions that make the consumptive man worse. They will also tell you that a bacillus is the cause of tuberculosis. But if the man had not been susceptible to the bacillus he could not have been affected by it. As a matter of fact, the tubercules come first and the bacillus is secondary. It has never been found prior to the tubercule, but it follows that, and comes then as a scavenger. The cause of the tubercular deposit rests with the psora, the chronic miasm. Bacilli are not the cause of disease, they never come until after the disease.

Allopaths are really taking the sequence for the consequence, thus leading to a false theory, the bacteria theory. You may destroy the bacteria and yet not destroy the disease. The susceptibility remains the same, and only those that are susceptible will take the disease. Bacteria have a use, for there is nothing in the whole world that does not have a use, and there is nothing sent on earth to destroy man. The bacteria theory would make it appear that the all-wise Creator has sent these micro-organisms here to make man sick. We see from this paragraph that Hahnemann did not adopt any such theory as bacteriology.

This subject will be taken up in these lectures and fully illustrated, but I might throw out a few hints to set you thinking until we come to it again. We know that a dissecting wound is very serious if the body dissected is recently dead, and this we would suppose to be due to some bacteria of wonderful power capable of establishing such a dreadful erysipelatous poisoning that would go into man's blood and strike him down with a sort of septicæmia. In truth, soon after death we have a ptomaine poison, the dead body poison, which is alkaloidal in character, but we do not yet discover the presence of bacteria. The poison is there, and if a man pricks himself while dissecting that body and does not take care of the wound he may have a serious illness and die. But if after the cadaver has remained some time and become infected with bacteria, the dissector pricks himself the wound is not dangerous.

The more bacteria the less poison. A typhoid stool when it first passes from the bowel has a very scanty allowance of bacteria, and yet it is very poisonous. But let it remain until it becomes black with bacteria and it is comparatively benign. Why does the poison not increase with the bacteria? You can potentize, as I have done, a portion of a tuberculous mass alive with tubercular bacilli, and after potentizing it, after being triturated with sugar of milk and mashed to a pulp, it will continue to manifest its symptoms in the most potent form. You can precipitate the purulent tubercular fluid in alcohol, precipitate the entire animal life and potentize the supernatant fluid until you have reached the thirtieth potency, and having potentized or attenuated it until no microbe can be found, yet, if administered to healthy man, it will establish the nature of the disease in the economy, which is prior to phthisis. Thus we have the cause of phthisis, not in the bacteria, but in the virus, which the bacteria are sent to destroy. Man lives longer with the bacteria than he would without them. If we could succeed today in putting a fluid into the economy that would destroy the bacteria that consumptive would soon die.

The study of disease as to fundamental cause and apparent cause is an important subject. We cannot study cause unless we have first understood government associated with law. Hence recall to your mind that the *law directs and experience confirms*. Law is nothing but an orderly state of government from centre to circumference, a government in which there is a head. You show me a company that has no captain and you show me a disorderly company. Order exists from the highest to the lowest from centre to circumference.

Now I have led up to the point where you may ask, Is it not disorder for man to settle what is true by the senses? Let us as homœopaths turn our lives, our thinking abilities and our scientific life into order that we may begin to turn the human race into order. Let us adopt the plan of thinking of things from their beginning and following them in a series to their conclusions. No man is authority, but principle and law are authority. If this cannot be seen there is no use of proceeding any further with the study of Homœopathy. If man cannot see this he cannot see the necessity of harmony from centre to circumference, of government which has one head, and hence it would be useless for him to study the human body for the purpose of applying medicine to it. It must be accepted in this form or it will not satisfy man, it will not sustain his expectation, it will not do what he expects it to do; it will only accomplish what Allopathy has accomplished, viz., the establishment of confusion upon the economy.

LECTURE VI

§ 6. THE UNPREJUDICED OBSERVER NOTES ONLY CHANGE OF STATE AS SHOWN BY SYMPTOMS

Paragraph 6. The unprejudiced observer—well aware of the futility of transcendental speculations which can receive no confirmation from experience—be his powers of penetration ever so great, takes note of nothing in every individual disease, except the changes in the health of the body and of the mind which can be perceived externally by means of the senses; that is to say, he notices only the deviations from the former healthy state of the now diseased individual, which are felt by the patient himself, remarked by those around him and observed by the physician. All these perceptible signs represent the disease in its whole extent, that is, together they form the true and only conceivable portrait of the disease.

The teaching of this paragraph is that the symptoms represent to the intelligent physician all there is to be known of the nature of a sickness, that these symptoms represent the state of disorder, that sickness is only a change of state and that all the physician has to do is correct the disordered state. Hahnemann, it seems, would say that it is great folly for a man to look into the organs themselves for the purpose of establishing a theory to find out whether the stomach makes the man sick, or whether the stomach makes the liver sick and such like. We can only end in theory as long as we think that way. So long as we set the mind to thinking about a man's organs and how these things are brought about we are in confusion, but not so when we meditate upon the symptoms of the sick man as fully representing the nature of the disease after these have been carefully written out.

Hahnemann starts out in this paragraph by speaking of "the unprejudiced observer." It would almost seem impossible to find at the present time one who could be thus described. All men are prejudiced. Man is fixed in his politics, fixed in his religion, fixed in his ideas of medicine, and because of his prejudice he cannot reason. You need only to talk to him a moment on these subjects and he will begin to tell you what he thinks; he will give his opinion, as if that had anything to do with it. Men of the present day cannot recognize law, and hence they are prejudiced; but when men have authority on which they can rest, then they can get rid of their prejudices. Suppose we have a large dictionary that we say is an authority on the spelling of words. If a club of one hundred and fifty men who bought that dictionary, and put it into a closet and say, "That is how we agree to spell," that is a recognition by these men that the book is authority. There would be henceforth no argument on the question of spelling. But if there were no authority one man would spell one way and another man in another way; there would be no standard of spelling. Such is the state of medicine at the present day, there is no standard authority. One book is authority in one school, and in another school they have another book, and so there is confusion.

Men cannot get rid of their prejudices until they settle upon and recognize authority. In Homœopathy the law and its principles must be accepted as authority. When we know these it is easy to accept them as authority, but seeing they are not known there is no authority and everybody is prejudiced. Men often ask, "Doctor, what are your theories as to Homœopathy? What are your theories of medicine?" I have no theories. It is a thing that is settled from doctrine and principle, and I know nothing of theory. A woman came into my office this morning and said, "Doctor, I have always been treated by the old school, but the doctors were unable to decide whether the liver made my stomach sick or the stomach made the liver sick." This is only confusion. No organ can make the body sick; man is prior to his organs; parts of the body can be removed and yet man will exist. There is no such thing as one organ making another sick. When we realize that the course of things is from centre to circumference we must admit that the stomach was caused to be in disorder from the centre, and that the liver was caused to be in disorder from the centre, but not that they made each other sick. One who has been taught such ideas cannot rid himself of them for a long time. It is a matter of years to get out of these whims and notions which we have imbibed from our inheritance. We cannot rid ourselves of confusion until we learn what confusion is.

In this paragraph Hahnemann does not speak of changes of tissue or changes in the organs, but changes of state. Man could see and feel tissue changes, but these do not represent to the intelligent physician the nature of disease or disease cause, they only indicate that because of the disorder within certain results have followed. The unprejudiced observer can see that pathology does not represent the nature of the disease, because numerous so-called diseases can present the same pathology and the same phenomena. The trouble is that there are so few unprejudiced observers. To get rid of our prejudices is one of the first things we must do in the study of Homœopathy. Therefore let me beg of you, while sitting in this room, to lay aside all that you have heretofore imagined or presumed, the whims and notions, and "what I thought about it," the things that you have learned from men and books, and only follow after law and principle, things that cannot deceive, cannot vary.

Even law will deceive if man is of prejudiced mind, because then he misreads the law and doctrine, and when things are called black they look to him white; every image is inverted in his prejudiced mind, because he realizes only with his senses, and sees with his eyes and feels with his fingers only the appearance of things, just as we say that the sun rises, judging from our eyes, although we know from our intelligence that it does not rise. If we believe our senses only we will accept all the notions of men. If the senses were invariable men would agree, but they are variable and no two men will agree in everything, for just as men's observations differ so different notions and theories will be established. We must try to get rid of the prejudices that we have been born with and educated into, so that we can examine the principles and doctrines of Homœopathy and seek to verify them. If you cannot put aside your prejudices the principles will be folly to you. The unprejudiced observer is the only true scientist.

"He perceives in each individual affection nothing but changes of state." The changes of state are such as are observed by the patient when he says he is forgetful, that his mind does not operate as it did, that he is often in a state of confusion, that when he attempts to deliver a sentence a part of it goes away from him, the idea passes away, or that he is becoming irritable, whereas he was pleasant, that he is becoming sad, whereas he was cheerful before, that there are changes in his affections, in his desires and aversions. These things relate to states: not to diseased tissues, but to a state of disorder or want of harmony. Dr. Fincke expresses it as "a distunement."

After the patient has related everything he can about his change of state, the physician may be aided by information from outsiders, from relatives who look upon the patient with goodwill, who wish him well. If the husband be sick it is well to get the wife's testimony. After the physician has written down all the information in accordance with the directions of § 85 for the taking of the case he then commences to observe as much as he can concerning the disorder, but more particularly those things which the patient would conceal, or cannot relate, or does not know. Many patients do not know that they are awkward, that they do peculiar and strange things in the doctor's office—things that they would not do in health, and these are evidences of change of state.

The physician also notes what he sees, notes odors, the sounds of organs, chest sounds, intensity of fever, by his hand or by a thermometer, etc., and when he has gone over this entire image, including everything that can represent the disease, he has secured all that is of real value to him.

What if there are changes in tissue present? There is nothing in the nature of diseased tissue to point to a remedy; it is only a result of disease. Suppose there is an abdominal tumor, or a tumor of the mammary gland, there is nothing in the fact that it is a tumor or in the aspect of the tumor that would lead you to the nature of the change of state. The things that you can see, i.e., the changes in the tissues, are of the least importance, but what you perceive in the patient himself, how he moves and acts, his functions and sensations, are manifestations of what is going on in the internal economy. A state of disorder represents its nature to man by signs and symptoms, and these are things to be prescribed upon.

Take a case which as yet has no pathological changes, no morbid anatomy, one that has only functional changes; the collection of signs and symptoms presents to the intelligent physician the nature of the state and he is clear as to the remedy. But if the patient does not receive that remedy, what will happen? The case will go on for a while, perhaps for two or three years, and when he returns to you on examination you will find that he has cavities in his lungs or an abscess in his liver, or albumin in the urine, etc. If it were the last, according to the old-fashioned notions and theories, you must now prescribe for Bright's disease; you would not think that remedy which you figured out two years before fitted his case perfectly then and is what he must have now. But he needed that remedy from his childhood, and you were able to figure it out from the symptoms of his change of state pure and simple, without tissue changes. Do you suppose because the disease has now progressed into tissue change, the organs are breaking down and the man is going to die, that this has changed that primitive state? The man needs the same course of treatment that he has needed from his babyhood. The same idea of his disease must prevail now that prevailed before he had the tissue changes. Bright's disease is not a disease, it is simply the ultimate or organic condition which has followed the progress of the original change of state. Under other circumstances that change of state might have affected his liver or his lungs.

Tissue changes do not indicate the remedy, and so as physicians we must learn to examine symptoms which are prior to morbid anatomy, to go back to the very beginning. Such a patient as I have described must be looked upon as when he was in the simple change of state before matters were complicated. Besides this, there is no manner of treatment for Bright's disease or any other organic change. Our remedies appeal to man before his state has changed into disease ultimates, and these remedies do not change because morbid anatomy has come on, they apply as much after tissue changes as before it. If we do not know what the beginnings are we cannot in an intelligent way treat the endings.

In a footnote Hahnemann says, "I know not therefore how it was possible for physicians at the sick-bed to allow themselves to suppose that, without most carefully attending to the symptoms and being guided by them in the treatment, they ought to seek and could discover only the hidden and unknown interior what there was to be cured in the disease, etc." The learned man in the old school today would say, "Oh, I do not care anything about your symptoms. I do not care if you are forgetful or irritable. If you do not sleep I will give you something to make you sleep. But I must sound your liver, for that is the cause of all your trouble, and I will prescribe for that." He supposes the liver is the cause of all the trouble, and believes that when that is corrected he has cured his patient. What a false idea! His mind is upon mere theory. It is common, when they do not know what has killed a man, to make a post-mortem in order to discover the cause, and by this they find out certain pathological conditions; but the aim of the physician is to discover in his patient that just these conditions are present.

It is true, on the other hand, that the post-mortem affords the physician the means for a general study of the results of disease, which I would not, under any circumstances, prevent. Indeed, there are times when I would strongly encourage the study of morbid anatomy. The physician cannot know too much about the endings of disease; he should become thoroughly acquainted with the tissues in all conditions; but to study these with the idea that he is going thereby to cure sick folks, or that the things he picks up at such times are going to be applied in making prescriptions, is a great folly. It is astonishing that physicians should expect to find out by post-mortem and examinations of organs what to do for sick folks.

Physical diagnosis is very important in its own place. By means of physical diagnosis the physician may find out the changes in organs, how far the disease has progressed, and determine if the patient is incurable. It is necessary also in supplying information to Boards of Health. It may also decide whether you should give curative or palliative treatments. But the study of pathology is a separate and distinct thing from the study of Materia Medica.

In many instances foolish examinations are made. In the colleges women are examined with the speculum before a symptom is given, and if the mucous membrane is red the patient gets Hamamelis, and so on in a routine way through five or six remedies which cover all the complaints of women. Half a dozen remedies constitute the armamentarium of many of the eminent gynæcologists. Such a practice as that does not cure, does not even benefit temporarily, it is simply an outrage. But bad though it is, perhaps it is not so great an outrage as is perpetrated when the physician imagines the disease is local, and that when he has cauterized it the woman is well, not realizing for one moment that these things come from a cause and that curing that cause should be his aim. Yet such is the teaching of the old school.

Now while the signs and symptoms are the only things that can tell the physician what the patient needs, and while those signs and symptoms relate to change of state and not to change of tissue, still there are signs that relate to tissue changes, and one who is acquainted with symptoms may consider these as indicating a change of state. For example, there are signs that indicate that pus is forming, there are appearances that will lead the experienced physician to know that the results of disease are coming; these are not valuable things in hunting for the remedy, but simply indicate certain conditions. The physician must learn to distinguish these from the symptoms that portray the state of the patient.

We are now prepared to see that if the patient is cured from cause to effect he must remain cured; that is, if the true inner disorder is turned into order he will remain cured, because this order, which is of the innermost, will cause to flow into order that which is of the outermost and finally the function of the body to become orderly. The vital order will cause tissue order, because the vital order extends into the very outermost of the tissues, and tissue government and order is a vital order; so if the cure is from cause to effect, or from within out, the patient will remain cured. In incurable cases the effects may be removed temporarily or palliated, but the patient himself has not been cured as to the cause, and owing to the fact that the patient cannot be cured the old changes will return and grow stronger because it is in the nature of chronic cases to increase or progress.

Certain results of disease which remain after the patient is cured can be removed if necessary, but it is not well to remove them before the patient is cured. If a patient has a disease of the foot bones after a bad injury and the foot cannot be cured, first cure the patient, and then if the foot is so clumsy and useless that he would rather have a wooden one remove the foot. If you have to deal with a worthless honey-combed kneejoint, first cure the patient and then if the knee can never be useful and the limb is cold and the muscles are flabby consider the question of replacing it with an artificial one. If the economy after being turned into health cannot cure the knee nothing that can be done to the knee can cure it, Do not say that the patient is sick because he has a white swelling, but that the white swelling is there because the patient is sick.

LECTURE VII

In a footnote to paragraph 7, Hahnemann writes:

It is not necessary to say that every intelligent physician would first remove this exciting or maintaining cause (*causa occasionalis*), where it exists; the indisposition thereupon generally ceases spontaneously.

You have, I believe, been led to conclude that there are apparent diseases, which are not diseases, but disturbed states that may be called *indispositions*. A psoric individual has his periods of indispositions from external causes, but these external causes do not inflict psora upon him. Such a patient may disorder his stomach from abusing it and thus create an indisposition. Indispositions from external causes mimic the miasms, *i.e.*, their group of symptoms is an imitation of a miasmatic manifestation, but the removal of the external cause is likely to restore the patient to health. Business failures, depressing tribulations, unrequited affection producing suffering in young girls, are apparent causes of disease, but in reality they are only exciting causes of indispositions. The active cause is within and the apparent cause of sickness is without. If man had no psora, no deep miasmatic influence within his economy, he would be able to throw off all these business cares, he would not become insane from business depression, and the young girl would not suffer so from love affairs. There would be an orderly state. The physician then must discriminate between the causes that are apparent or external, the grosser things, from the truer causes of disease, which are from centre to circumference. In every instance where Hahnemann speaks of true sickness, he speaks of it as a miasmatic disease, but here he employs another word. "Then the *indisposition* usually yields of itself," or if the psoric condition has been somewhat disturbed, order can be restored by a few doses of the homœopathic remedy. To illustrate, if a man has disordered his stomach it will right itself on his ceasing to abuse it; but, if the trouble seems somewhat prolonged, a dose of medicine, like *Nux vomica* or whatever remedy is indicated, will help the stomach to right itself, and so long as he lives in an orderly way he will cease to feel this indisposition.

"The physician will remove from the room strong smelling flowers which have a tendency to cause syncope and hysterical sufferings." There are some nervous girls who are so sensitive to flowers that they will faint from the odor. There are other individuals who are so psoric in their nature that they cannot live in the ordinary atmosphere; some must be sent to the mountains, some to warm lands, some to cold lands. This is removing the occasioning cause, the apparent aggravating cause of suffering. A consumptive in the advanced stages, one who is steadily running down in Philadelphia, must be sent to a climate where he can be made comfortable. The external or apparent cause, the disturbing cause in his sick state, is thus removed but the cause of his sickness is prior to this. The physician does not send the patient away for the purpose of curing him, but for the purpose of making him comfortable. "He will extract from the cornea the foreign body that excites inflammation of the eye, loosen the overtight bandage on a wounded limb that threatens to cause mortification, lay bare and put a ligature on the wounded artery that produces fainting, endeavour to promote the expulsion by vomiting of belladonna berries, etc., that may have been swallowed. Now, without the circumstances and surroundings in which Hahnemann stated these things, it has been asserted in the public prints that Hahnemann advised emetics. A class of so-called physicians have taken this note of Hahnemann's for a cloak as a means of covering up their scientific rascality, their use of external applications. They tell us Hahnemann said so, but we see it becomes a lie.

Here is another note: "In all times, the old school physicians, not knowing how else to give relief, have sought to combat and if possible to suppress by medicines, here and there a *single* symptom from among a number in diseases." This course of singling out a group of symptoms, and treating that group alone as the disease is incorrect, because it has no due relation to the entirety of the man. A group of symptoms may arise through the uterus and vagina, and one who is of this understanding has a plan for removing only the group of symptoms that belong to his speciality, whereby he thinks he has eradicated the trouble. Hahnemann condemns this doctrine, and we see at once its great folly. In many instances there are, at the same time, manifestations of "heart disease," "liver disease," etc. (that is, speaking in their terms; these are not diseases at all, as we know), so that every specialist might be consulted, and each one would direct the assault at his own particular region, and so the patient goes the rounds of all the specialists and the poor man dies. An old allopathic physician once made the remark about a case of pneumonia that he was treating, that he had broken up the pneumonia. "Yes," said another physician, "the pneumonia is cured, but the patient is going to die." That is the way when one of these groups of symptoms is removed; constipation may be removed by physic; liver symptoms may sometimes be removed temporarily by a big dose of calomel; ulcers can be so stimulated that they will heal up; but the patient is not cured. Hahnemann says it is strange that the physician cannot see that the removal of these symptoms is not followed by cure, that the patient is worse off for it.

Some patients are not sufficiently ill to see immediately the bad consequences of the closure of a fistulous opening but if a patient is threatened with phthisis, or is a weakly patient, the closure of that fistulous opening of the anus will throw him into a flame of excitement and will cause his death in a year or two. The more rugged ones will live a number of years before they break down, and they are held up as evidences of cure. Such treatment is not based upon principles, and close observation will convince a thoughtful man of its uselessness and danger. The fistulous opening came there because it was of use, and probably if it had been permitted to exist would have remained as a vent until the patient was cured. When the patient is cured the fistulous opening ceases to be of use, the necessity for it to remain open has ceased, and it heals up of itself.

The *Organon* condemns on principle the removal of external manifestations of disease by an external means whatever. A psoric case is one in which there is no external or traumatic cause. The patient perhaps has the habit of living as nearly an orderly life as it is possible for anyone to assume at the present day, going the regular rounds of service, using coffee and tea not at all or only in small quantity, careful in diet, removing all external things which are the causes of indispositions, and yet this patient remains sick. The signs and symptoms that are manifested are the true impress of nature, they constitute the outwardly reflected image of the inward nature of the sickness. "Now as in a disease from which no manifest exciting or maintaining cause has to be removed we can perceive nothing but the morbid symptoms, it must be the symptoms alone by which the disease demands and points to the remedy suited to relieve it."

Hahnemann's teaching is that there is a use in this symptom image, and that every curable disease presents itself to the intelligent physician in the signs and symptoms that he can perceive. In viewing a long array of symptoms an image is presented to the mind of an internal disorder, and this is all that the intelligent physician can rely upon for the purpose of cure.

This divides Homœopathy into two parts, the science of Homœopathy and the art of Homœopathy. The science treats of the knowledges relating to the doctrines of cure, the knowledge of principle or order, which you may say is physiology; the knowledge of disorder in the human economy, which is pathology (that is, the science of disease, not morbid anatomy), and the knowledge of cure. The science of Homœopathy is first to be learned to prepare one for the application of that science, which is the art of Homœopathy. If we cast our eyes over those who have been taught, self-taught or otherwise, we see that some can learn the science, become quite famous and pass excellent examinations, and are utterly unable to apply the science, or, in other words, to practice the art of healing, for all healing consists in making application of the science.

We study disease as a disorder of the human economy in the symptoms of the disease itself. We also study disease from the symptoms of medicines that have caused disorder in the economy. Indeed, we can study the nature and quality of disease as much by studying the Materia Medica as by studying symptoms of disease, and when we cannot fill our time in studying symptoms from sick folks it is well to use the time in studying the symptomatology of the Materia Medica. True knowledge consists in becoming acquainted with and understanding the nature and quality of a remedy, its appearance, its image and its relation to man in his sickness; then by studying the nature of sickness in the human family to compare that sickness with symptoms of the Materia Medica. By this means we become acquainted with the law of cure and all that it leads to, and formulate doctrines by which the law may be applied and made use of, by arranging the truth in form to be perceived by the human mind.

This is but the science and we may, notwithstanding, fail to heal the sick. You will observe some, who know the science, go out and make improper application of the remedies, and seem to have no ability to perceive in a remedy that which is similar to a disease. I believe if they had a candid love for the work they would overcome this, but they think more of their pocket books. The physician who is the most successful is he who will first heal for the love of healing, who will practice first for the purpose of verifying his knowledge and performing his use for the love of it. I have never known such a one to fail. This love stimulates him to proceed and not to be discouraged with his first failures, and leads him to success, in simple things first and then in greater things. If he did not have an unusual affection for it he would not succeed in it. An artist once was asked how it was that he mixed his paints so wonderfully, and he replied, "With brains, sir." So one may have all the knowledge of Homœopathy that it is possible for a human being to have, and yet be a failure in applying that art in its beauty and loveliness. If he have no affection for it, it will be seen to be a mere matter of memory and superficial intelligence. As he learns to love it, and dwell upon it as the very life of him, then he understands it as art and can apply it in the highest degree. The continuous application of it will lead any physician of ordinary intelligence so far into the perception of his work that he will be able to perceive by the symptoms the whole state of the economy, and when reading provings to perceive the very nature of the sickness expressed in the provings. This degree of perception will enable him to see the "outwardly reflected image." You will not have to observe long, or be among physicians long, before you will find that many of them have a most external memory of the Materia Medica, that they have no idea of the nature of medicines they use, no perception of the quality or image of a remedy. It does not come up before their mind as an artist's picture; it is cold, it is far away. An artist works on a picture so that he sees it day and night, he figures it out from his very affections, he figures out every line that he is going to put in the next day, stands before it and he is delighted in it and loves it. So it is with the image of a remedy. That image comes out before the mind so that it is the outwardly reflected image of the inner nature, as if one man had proved it. If the symptoms do not take form the physician does not know his patient and does not know his remedy. This is not a thing that can open out to the mind instantly. You are, as it

were, coming out of a world where the education consists in
memorizing symptoms or memorizing key-notes or learning prescriptions, with really nothing in the mind, and the memory is only
charged with a mass of information that has no application, and is
only confusion leading man to worse confusion. There is no order
in it. Hahnemann says: "In a word, the totality of the symptoms
must be the principal, indeed the only thing the physician has to
take note of in every case of disease, and to remove by means of
his art, in order that it shall be cured and transformed into health."
That is the turning of internal disorder into order manifested in
the way we have heretofore explained, viz., from above downward,
from within out and in the reverse order of the coming of the
symptoms.

LECTURE VIII

ON SIMPLE SUBSTANCE

§ 9. In the healthy condition of man, the spiritual vital force, the dynamis that animates the material body, rules with unbounded sway, and retains all parts of the organism in admirable, harmonious, vital operation, as regards both sensations and functions, so that our indwelling, reason-gifted mind can freely employ this living healthy instrument for the higher purposes of our existence.

This paragraph introduces the vital principle. It would hardly seem possible that Hahnemann, in the time he lived, could say so much in a few lines. In the seventh section of the first edition of the *Organon*, Hahnemann wrote: "There must exist in the medicine a healing principle; the understanding has a presentiment of it," but after the *Organon* had gone through a number of editions Hahnemann had somewhat changed, and in this work, which is the 1883 edition, he distinctly calls a unit of action in the whole organism the vital force. You get the idea from some of his expressions that the harmony itself is a force, but I do not think that Hahnemann intends to teach that way. We cannot consider the vital principle as harmony, nor harmony as principle; principle is something that is prior to harmony. Harmony is the result of principle or law.

Hahnemann could perceive this immaterial vital principle. It was something he arrived at himself, from his own process of thinking. There was paucity of individual ideas at that time, *i.e.*, ideas outside of the accepted sciences, but Hahnemann thought much, and by thinking he arrived at the idea contained in this paragraph, which only appears in the last edition, "In the healthy condition of man the *immaterial vital principle* animates the material body." If he had used the words "immaterial vital substance," it would have been even stronger, for you will see it to be true that it is a substance.

At the present day advanced thinkers are speaking of *the fourth state of matter* which is *immaterial substance*. We now say the

solids, liquids and gases and the radiant form of matter. Substance
in simple form is just as positively substance as matter in concrete
form. The question then comes up for consideration and study:
What is the vital force? What is its character, quality or *esse* ? Is
it true that man only has this vital force? Is it possessed by no
animal, no mineral? For a number of years there has been a continuous discussion of force as force, or power to construct. The
thought that force has nothing prior to it leads man's mind into
insanity. If man can think of energy as something substantial he can
better think of something substantial as having energy. When he
thinks of something that has essence, has actual being, he must think
of that *esse* as something existing and as having something which
has ultimates. He must think in a series whereby cause enters into
effect and furthermore into a series of effects. If he do not do this
he destroys the very nature and idea of influx and continuance. If
man does not know what is continuous, if he does not realize that
there are beginnings, intermediates and ends, he cannot think, for
the very foundation of thought is destroyed.

What do we mean by influx? As a broad and substantial illustration let us think of a chain. What is it that holds the last link
of a chain to its investment or first attachment? At once we will
say the intermediate link. What is it that connects that link? Its
previous link, and so on to the first link and its attachment. Do we
not thus see that there is one continuous dependence from the last
to the first hook? Wherever that chain is separated it is as much
separated as possible, and there is no longer influx from one link
to the other. In the same way as soon as we commence to think of
things disconnectedly we lose the power of communication between
them. All things must be united or the series is broken and influx
ceases.

Again, we see that man exists as to his body, but as yet we do
not see all the finer purposes of his being.

To believe that man exists without a cause, to believe that his
life force goes on for a while and does not exist from something
prior to it, to think that there is not constantly and continuously
that influx from cause whereby he continues to live, demontrates
that the man who does so is an irrational being. From his senses
man has never been able to prove that anything can exist except
it has continually flowing into it that which holds it in continuance.
Then why should he, when he goes into the immaterial world,

assume that energy is the first? We shall find by a continued examination of the question of simple substance that we have some reason for saying that energy is not energy *per se*, but that it is a powerful substance, and is endowed from intelligence that is of itself a substance.

The materialist to be consistent with his principles is obliged to deny the soul, and to deny a substantial God, because the energy which he dwells upon so much is nothing, and he must assume that God is nothing, and therefore there is none. But the one who is rational will be led to see that there is a supreme God, that He is substantial, that He is a substance. Everything proceeds from him and the whole series from the supreme to the most ultimate matter in this way is connected. Just as surely as there is a separation, and not a continuous influx from first to last, ultimates will cease to exist.

The true holding together of the material world is performed by the simple substance. There are two worlds that come apparently to the mind of man, the world of thought and the world of matter; that is, the world of immaterial substance and the world of material substance. The world of material substance is in order and harmony. Everything that appears before the eye has beginnings. The forms are harmonious; every crystal of a metal crystallizes in accordance with order; man's very anatomy forms harmoniously. We see nothing in the material world to account for this, but we perceive that all things are held in position because of the continuous influx from first to last. There is no break in the chain and no break in the flow of power from first to last. Nothing can exist unless its cause be inflowing into it continuously. We see that all things made by man's hand decay and fall to pieces in time, but look at the things perpetuated from influx, look at their order and harmony from time to eternity, working by the same plan and in the same order.

There are many qualities predicated of simple substance, and one of the first propositions we have to consider is that simple substance is *endowed with formative intelligence, i.e.,* it intelligently operates and forms the economy of the whole animal, vegetable and mineral kingdoms. Everything with form goes on its natural course and assumes and continues its own private state. The laws of chemistry by analysis may be so revealed to man that he can detect all elements because they conduct themselves uniformly. The simple substance gives to everything its own type of life, gives it distinction, gives it identity whereby it differs from all other things. The crystal of the earth has its own association, its own identity; it is endowed with a simple substance that will establish its identity from everything in the animal kingdom, everything in the mineral kingdom. This is due to the formative intelligence of simple substance, which is continuous from its beginning to its end. If we examine the frost work upon the window we see its tendency to manifest formative intelligence. Plants grow in fixed forms. So it is with man from his beginning to his end; there is continuous influx into man from his cause. Hence man and all forms are subject to the laws of influx. If man is in the highest order and is rational, he wills to keep himself in continuous order, that his thoughts may continue rational; but he is so placed in freedom that he can also destroy his rationality.

This substance is *subject to changes;* in other words, it may be flowing in order or disorder, may be sick or normal; and the changes to a great extent may be observed or even created by man himself. Man may cause it to flow in disorder.

Any simple substance may *pervade the entire material substance without disturbing or replacing it.* Magnetism may occupy a substance and not displace any of it nor cause derangement of its particles or crystals. Cohesion is a simple substance; it is not the purpose of cohesion to disturb or displace the substance that it occupies. Therefore this first substance, or primitive substance, exists as such in all distinct forms of growths of concrete forms, and the material, concrete, individual entity is not disturbed or displaced by the simple substance; the simple substance is capable of occupying the material substance without accident to that substance or to itself.

When the simple substance is an active substance it *dominates and controls the body it occupies.* It is the cause of force. The body does not move, think or act unless it has its interior degrees of immaterial substance, which acts upon the economy continuously in the most beautiful manner, but as soon as the body is separated from its characterizing simple substance there is a cessation of influx. The energy derived from the simple substance keeps all things in order. By it are kept in order all functions, and the perpetuation of the forms and proportions of every animal, plant and mineral. All operation that is possible is due to the simple substance, and by it the very universe itself is kept in order. It not only operates every material substance, but it is the cause of co-operation of all things.

Examine the universe and behold the stars, the sun and the moon; they do not interfere with each other, they are kept in continuous order. Everything is in harmony and is kept so by the simple substance. We see co-operation in every degree, and this co-operation working in perfect harmony; we see human beings moving about; we see things going on about us on the earth; we see the trees of the forest making room for each other, existing in perfect harmony; the very sounds of the forest have harmony; and all this co-ordination is brought about by the simple substance. There is nothing more wonderful than the co-ordination of man's economy, his will and his understanding and his movements, which co-ordination is carried on by the life substance. Without this all matter is dead and cannot be used for the higher purposes of its existence. By the aid of simple substance the Divine Creator is able to use all created beings and forms for their highest purpose.

Matter is subject to reduction, and it can be continuously reduced until it is in the form of simple substance, *but it is not subject to restitution.* No substance can be returned to its ultimate form after it has been reduced to its primitive form. It is not in the power of man to change from first to last; that is, it is not in his power to ultimate the simple substance. This is retained for the Supreme Power Himself, from whom power continually flows through all the primitive substance to the end; *i.e.,* to ultimates. Now do you begin to see that the thing that does not start from its beginning with a purpose is not a thing, or, to put it another way, what makes anything a thing is because of its purpose or ultimate which is use, and there is never created a thing without a purpose. If it does not exist in continuous series from first to last it cannot be of use or of purpose; hence the end is in the first, and the end is in every succeeding link to its ultimate, the very form in which the use is to be appropriated and established. When you establish the first link in the chain you have the end of the next link in view.

The simple substances may exist as *simple, compound* or *complex,* and as such never disturb harmony, but always continue from first to last, and in that way all purposes are conserved. Throughout chemistry we can observe this compounding. We find

Iodine uniting with its base; *i.e.*, two simple substances compounding in keeping, with their own individual plan, realiably and intelligently in accordance with the affinities for each other. When substances come together in that way they do not disturb the simple substance of each other, there is nothing destroyed, each one retains its own identity, and they can be reduced again to their simples by reaction and reagents. Now all of these enter into the human body and every element in the human body preserves its identity throughout and wherever found can be identified. Such combination, however, merely represents a composite state. But when these composite substances and simple substances are brought into an additional condition; *i.e.*, when they are presided over and dominated by something they may be said to enter into a very *complex* form, and in the body a life force keeps every other force in order. Dynamic simple substances often dominate each other in proportion to their purpose, one having a higher purpose than another. This vital force, which is a simple substance, is again dominated by another simple substance still higher, which is the soul. It has been the aim of a great many philosophers by study to arrive at some conclusion concerning the soul. They have attempted to locate it 'at some particular point, but we can see from the above that it is not in circumscribed location.

In considering simple substance we cannot think of time, place or space, because we are not in the realm of mathematics nor the restricted measurements of the world of space and time, we are in the realm of simple substance. It is only finite to think of place and time. *Quantity* cannot be predicated of simple substance, *only quality in degrees of fineness.* We will see the importance of this in its special relation to Homœopathy, by using an illustration. When you have administered *Sulphur* 55 m. in infrequent doses and find it will not work any longer you give the *c.m.* potency and see the curative action taken up at once. Do we not see by this that we have entered a new series of degrees and are dealing entirely with quality?

The simple substance also has *adaptation.* At this point man's reasoning comes up, leading to false conclusions from appearances, so that he has accepted what is called the environment theory. That the individual has an adaptation to his environment is not questioned, but what is it that adapts itself to environment? The dead body cannot. When we reason from within out we see that the simple substance adapts itself to its surroundings, and tends to adapt its house to the surroundings, and thus the human body is kept in a state of order, in the cold or in the heat, in the wet and damp, and under all circumstances. The surroundings themselves produce nothing, are not causes, they are only circumstances.

The life substance within the body is the vice-regent of the soul, and the soul in turn is also a simple substance. All that there is of the soul operates and exists within every part of the human body, and thus it is that simple substance acts as a vital force. The soul adapts the human body to all its purposes, the higher purposes of its being. The simple substance when it exists in the living human body keeps that body animated, keeps it moving, perfects its uses, superintends all parts and at the same time keeps the operation of mind and will in order. Let any disturbance occur in the vital substance and we see how suddenly inco-ordination will come. There is harmonious co-operation when the vital substance is continued in its normal quality; that is, in health what is more perfect than the human body in health, and what evidence have we of any greater wreck than the human body when it is not in health?

We see also that this vital substance when in a natural state, when in contact with the human body, is *constructive;* it keeps the body continuously constructed and reconstructed. But when the opposite is true, when the vital force from any cause withdraws from the body, we see that the forces that are in the body being turned loose are destructive. When these forces are not dominated and controlled by the vital force the body tends to decay at once. So we see that the vital force is constructive or formative, and in its absence there is death and destruction. If we examine the very simplest form of living organism, the plasson body, we will observe that it has the essentials of life, has everything in it that the very highest order of life has; it has the properties and qualities of the life substance of man and animals; it reproduces itself, it moves, it feeds, it is endowed with influx, and, lastly, it can be killed. Now when you have said these things, you have predicated much of the vital substance, or the highest and of the lowest. It asserts its identity; it moves and feeds; it propagates and can be killed. It does not sustain its identity by chemical analysis, because when it is chemically analyzed it is no longer protoplasm. Protoplasm is only protoplasm when it is living. Chemically, all there is to be found of protoplasm is C.O.H.N. and S., but the life substance cannot be found. You put together 54 parts of C., 21 of O., 16 of N., 7 of H., and 2 of S., and what do you suppose you will have? Simply a composite something, but not that complexity which we identify as protoplasm. In analyzing the protoplasm, what has become of the life force? There is no difference in weight after death; the simple substance cannot be weighed. Neither weight, time nor space can be predicated of the simple substance; and it is not subject to the physical laws, such as gravitation.

Now, when we consider this substance as an energy, a force, or dynamis,—that is, something possessing power,—the subject is intelligible. Inert elements have in their nature not only their own identifying simple substance, but they have *degrees* of this identifying simple substance. The human body also has its degrees of life substance, existing in degrees suitable for all its uses. The innermost degrees of life substances are suitable to the will and understanding, the outermost degrees to the very coarsest tissue, and there is one continuous series of quality, in degrees from the innermost to the outermost. Every cell has within it the innermost and the outermost, because there is nothing in that which is coarsest but has that which is finest, too. The outermost envelopes are dominated by the coarser degrees of simple substance, and the innermost qualities are dominated by the innermost degrees. Each portion has an appropriate form, and from. the outermost to the innermost it has all. Otherwise the human body could not be dominated or ruled by the soul. Each tissue has within it its portion of the vital substance, each having its own peculiar kind of function. Inert substances have their own degrees. *Silica* has its degrees of simple substance within it, which can be brought out by the process of potentization, whereby it may be continuously simplified, rendered finer and finer, so that each portion which remains may, by continued potentization, be adapted to the higher degrees of the simple substance of man. The thirtieth potency of *Silica* will be sufficiently similar in form to reach in a curative way some of the diseases of man, viz., such as are dominating his economy in a correspondingly superficial and coarse series of the body. But it is true that *Silica* ceases after a time to act in the thirtieth potency, and it has to be further potentized in order that it may be similar in quality to the inner degrees, even until it reaches the very innermost or finest degrees of the simple substance.

Everything in the universe has its aura or atmosphere. Every star and planet has an atmosphere. The sun's atmosphere is its light and heat. Every human being has his atmosphere or aura; every animal has its atmosphere or aura. This aura is present in all entities. What may be said to be the aura of musk? That is a strong physical aura which almost everyone can perceive. A grain of musk has been kept for experiment's sake, in a bottle for seventeen years, giving off a perceptible aura yet without loss of weight. As a further evidence of aura, take, for instance, the animals which prey upon their food and you know that they can discover by an extremely intense aura states that man cannot discover. This is not an ordinary nose, but it is really the very instinct of the animal, whereby he perceives what is prey. His instinct is analogous to man's perception, and by this instinct he discovers his prey, when man would not be able to discover it. Man can discover musk in a bottle, but it is doubtful if man could discover the finest aura by its odor. This aura becomes useful and introduces a prominent sphere in the study of homœopathics.

The consciousness between two simple substances is really that atmosphere by which one knows the other, and by which all affinities and repulsions between simple substances are known. They are in harmony or in antagonism. Human beings are thus classified by positives and negatives. Minerals and the world generally are classified by positives and negatives. This has an underlying cause. Substances are extremely powerful when meeting other substances that are antagonistic in any way, and also when meeting substances in a destructive way. The formative processes are often brought about by destruction; forms are destroyed in order that new forms may exist, and new forms therefore are often created from simple substance.

There are two realms or worlds, the realm or world of cause and the realm or world of ultimates. In this outermost or physical world we can see only with the eye, touch with the finger, smell with the nose, hear with the ear; such is the realm of results. The world of cause is invisible, is not discoverable by the five senses; it is the world of thought and discoverable only by the understanding. That which we see about us is only the world of ends, but the world of cause is invisible. It is possible that we may perceive the innermost, and it is important also that man may know and look from within upon all things in the physical world, instead of starting in the physical world and attempting to look upon things in the immaterial world. He will then account for law and perceive the operation of law. Homœopathy exists as law; its causes are in the realm of causes. If it did not exist in the world of causes it could not exist in the world of ultimates. It is in the realm of cause that we must look for the primaries in the study of Homœopathy.

Of course it will be seen that the whole of this subject looks toward the establishment of a new system of pathology, which will be the groundwork of Homœopathy. All disease causes are in simple substance; there is no disease cause in concrete substance considered apart from simple substance. We therefore study simple substance, in order that we may arrive at the *nature* of sick-making substances. We also potentize our medicines in order to arrive at their simple substance; that is, at the nature and quality of the remedy itself. The remedy to be homœopathic must be similar in quality and similar in *action* to disease cause.

LECTURE IX

Organon § 10. The material organism, without the vital force, is capable of no sensation, no function, no self-preservation; it derives all sensation and performs all the functions of life solely by means of the immaterial being (the vital force) which animates the material organism in health and in disease. § 11. When a person falls ill it is only this spiritual, self-acting (automatic) vital force, everywhere present in his organism, that is primarily deranged by the dynamic influence upon it of a morbific agent inimical to life; it is only the vital force, deranged to such an abnormal state, that can furnish the organism with its disagreeable sensations and incline it to the irregular processes which we call disease; for, as a power invisible in itself, and only cognizable by the effects on the organism, its morbid derangement only makes itself known by the manifestation of disease in the sensations and functions of those parts of the organism exposed to the senses of the observer and physician; that is, by *morbid symptoms,* and in no other way can it make itself known.

It is clear that Hahnemann wishes to teach that it is a disorder of the activities of the internal man, a lack of harmony or lack of balance, which gives forth the signs and symptoms by which we recognize disease. These sensations constitute the language of disorder; *i.e.,* the means by which we recognize disorder and disease. This immaterial vital principle, this simple substance, everywhere pervades the organism, and in disease this disorder everywhere pervades the organism, it pervades every cell and every portion of the human economy. We will see in course of time that the change in form of a cell is the result first of disorder, that the derangement of the immaterial vital principle is the very beginning of the disorder, and that with this beginning there are changes in sensation by which man may know this beginning, which occurs long before there is any visible change in the material substance of the body.

The patient himself can feel by his sensations the changes, and this is inimical to life, and death immediately follows, for life in its fullest sense is freedom. As soon as the internal economy is deprived in any manner of its freedom, death is threatening; where freedom is lost death is sure to follow.

So it is when there is the inflowing of a simple substance that has the form or essence of a disease. It is in its essence an evil that is flowing into the economy, but it is a simple substance. Everything is substantial or real, and has in itself operating and perpetuating power. The fact that it can operate and perpetuate is the evidence of power, and if it has power it results in something. Every cause of disease then has form. If it were not in the form of single substance it could not affect the forms of simple substance in the natural state of the economy. Moreover, it has its association, from the finest forms of physical substance to the crudest, from beginning to end, from the inner to the outer. Such changes and activities as result in the very crudest forms are but the results of disease through a series of degrees, coarser and coarser to the outermost man. Everything that can be seen, that can be observed with the aid of the finest instrument, is but the result. Nothing in the world of immaterial substance can be seen with any faculty that is capable of seeing things in the world of material substance. The employment of instruments of precision will enable us to see the finest disease results, which are the outcome or results of things immaterial, the bacteria for instance, the very finest form of animal or vegetable life; but the cause of disease is a million times more subtle than these and cannot be seen by the human eye. The finest visible objects are but results of things still finer, so that the cause rests within. The morbific agents that Hahnemann refers to are simply the extremely fine forms of simple substance, or to bring them down to human thought we might call them viruses; but viruses are often gross because they can sometimes be observed by the vision of man, and therefore we must remember that within the virus is its innermost and that this innermost is in itself capable of giving form to the outermost, which is the visible virus aggregated and concentrated.

The coarser forms would be comparatively harmless were it not for their interiors. Disease products are comparatively harmless were it not for the fact that they contain an innermost and it is the innermost itself that is causative. The bacteria are the result of conditions within, they are, as it were, evolved by a spontaneous generation—literally, that is what it is. Every virus is capable of assuming forms and shapes in ultimates. The causes of ultimates are not from without but the immaterial invisible center. Those things that appear to man's eye are evolved, just as man himself is formed from a center which has the power of evolving, an endowment from the Creator, operating under fixed general laws.

It is only when the vital principle is disturbed by cause of a disease character (that is the innermost of a virus in the form of a simple substance) that it gives forth any consciousness of itself. If there were no disturbing influence in the interiors of man he never would have symptoms. As you sit there in your seats in a perfect state of quietude or tranquility you are not conscious of your eyes, of your limbs, of your hair. You have to stop and think whether you feel or not. When all the functions are carried on in a perfectly orderly way you have no consciousness of your body, which means that you are in freedom. When not in freedom the individual says. "I feel." It is this disturbance of an invisible character which comes from cause, and appears by changes in the activities of the body, changes in sensations, changes in functions. It is in accordance with all-wise Providence that these sensations should appear to the physician who shall be intelligent enough to read them and know what they mean. They are a warning, they are for us, for purpose. No feeling a man can have is without purpose, as there is nothing in the universe without its use. Hence these morbid sensations reveal to the physician that there is disorder.

To establish freedom should be the aim of the physician, and if a physician's work does not result in placing his patient in freedom he cannot heal the sick, for healing the sick is placing the patient in freedom, giving him absolute physical freedom. If the physician causes the pains to cease by a dose of Morphine, can we call that freedom? Is the patient not made stupid beyond the recognition of the nature of his feelings? The large doses of the old school produce anything but freedom. We must look elsewhere to find that kind of healing which turns disorder into order and makes man free. By removing the signs and symptoms in an orderly way, by converting disorder into order so that the symptoms no longer have a cause (for as we have already seen when the economy is turned into order it ceases to give forth symptoms), we place our patients in freedom, both physical and mental.

"Only the vital principle thus disturbed can give to the organism its abnormal sensations and incline it to the irregular actions we call disease." This is totally different from calling the results of disease the disease, e.g., calling Bright's disease, cancer, or palsy, diseases. Most of the conditions of the human economy that are called diseases in the books are not diseases, but the results of disease. To call a group of symptoms a disease of one part, and another group of symptoms a disease of another part, is a great heresy and leads to errors in prescribing that can never be corrected. Organic change is the result of disease.

Morbid disturbances can be perceived solely by means of the expression of disease in the sensations and actions! We would have no means of perceiving the morbid disturbance of the invisible principle except by morbid sensations, and if these were not present we would have no means of putting the patient in freedom. There are patients so sick that they cannot be put in freedom, those for whom there are no means of cure, and in these, while the internal structural changes are going on slowly, the morbid symptoms are not present. Such patients continually change doctors and change climates, recognizing, as it were, that no one is capable of relieving them. With an incurable change in a vital organ, all or most of the symptoms that existed go away; the symptoms of the diseases are suppressed, as it were, by the tremendous strain upon the system.

This is particularly true of the malignant forms of disease results. The symptoms that existed years ago have disappeared and the patient says "Oh, they did not amount to anything; I had had them all my life." But those are the symptoms that would manifest to the physician the nature of the remedy, for they give to him the real image of the sickness.

Some doctors say: "Oh, we will have a remedy for cancer some day," having in mind only the symptoms of cancer; that is, the symptoms that represent the results of disease and not the symptoms that represent the disease itself. There is a vast difference between these two. These physicians would not talk so if they only knew and would only think in this proper and wholesome fashion, that to cure the patient would be to cure the cancer, and in order to cure the patient it is necessary to go back in his history and get those symptoms that represent the patient in a state of disease and not the tissues in a state of disease results. In the latter state, the original symptoms of the disease have often disappeared; they are, as it were, swallowed up. So it is when the innermost disease has acted and the whole body is full of disease results, such as dropsical conditions, or pus sacs, or hip-joint abscesses. The pains make the patient unable to think of his symptoms. Then these physicians come along and prescribe for the resultant states and end in failure.

They give *Silica* for hip-joint disease and *Bufo* for epilepsy, and so on, giving medicines for groups of symptoms.

That is not Homœopathy. Such men then go off and say: "Oh, I have tried everything," but they have tried nothing but modern practice. It is a travesty upon Homœopathy. The expert physician can listen to signs and symptoms before morbid changes have taken place, and if no medicines have ever been administered, if no drugging has been resorted to, no morphine and no other violent and vicious drugs, the image stands out before him in relief; it is perfect, because it has not been meddled with. It speaks with clearness, and the physician who is intelligent can learn to read it. But the physician who is not capable of seeing that this is different from the group of pathological symptoms that represent the so-called fixed diseases, if he cannot make a distinction between the symptoms that represent the disease *per se* and the symptoms that represent the result of disease, he will never practice Homœopathy successfully. If he cannot understand it he had better work at it until he does understand it; he must continue to labour until he can discriminate between the organic symptoms associated with the results of disease and the pure signs given forth by nature. Every few days I run across a homœopathic physician who asks: "What remedy are you using in such and such case?" Such a thing has no place in my mind, and I look upon one who speaks in that way as a man untrained in homœopathics. I truly have lost my patience over such things, for the old gray-heads, who have practiced for years and pretended to practice Homœopathy, do not hesitate to say that "the best remedy for epilepsy" is so and so.

What nonsense! That is not adjusting the remedy to the state of the patient that existed before he had these structural changes and fixed groups of symptoms, for if you adjust a remedy to the pathological condition you are not adjusting it to the patient, to his very beginnings down to the present time. He need not have pathological results, all he needs to have is symptoms. The patient can cure his own morbid anatomy. If you will take away the first state of disorder his economy will be safe. If the results of disease cannot be removed the patient himself will return to health and the morbid anatomy will undergo such changes that it will not affect his state of health. The fibrinous adhesions needs not necessarily go away a state of quiescence comes and remains year after year so long as he remains well.

To think of remedies for cancer is confusion, but to think of remedies for the patient who appears to have cancer is orderly, and you will be astonished to know what wonderful changes will take place in these conditions when remedies that correspond to the conditions before the cancer began are administered. Cancer is the result of disorder, which disorder must be turned in order and must be healed. We dwell upon this, for many paragraphs bring out this distinction between symptoms and results of disease. The true morbid sensations of a healthy organism are what we must first consider. It is first assumed that the organism is in a state of health and capable of performing its functions, and then the morbid sensations of this healthy organism are the symptoms that come to the physician as a forerunner of death in parts, and finally death of the whole. The patient tells the physician his sensations, of the numbness of his fingers, of the pricking in his skin, of the pain in his stomach, etc., all the sensations of any part of which he is reminded. The healthy man is not reminded of his parts. He passes his stool without pain in the part. If he has pain or bleeding he is reminded of this part. If he passes his urine without sensation we say it is normal and he is in freedom, but if burning and smarting and tenesmus follow he is reminded of it, and these sensations constitute symptoms.

If the patient is waxy and pallid, has papules and pustules, or swollen and varicose veins with red face, red eyes, etc., these the physician can see and note down. Again there are things that the physician cannot see and that the patient cannot tell, that the mother, sister, husband or wife should relate to the physician at his office. These symptoms constitute what there is knowable of the sickness, that which appears to the mind of the physician upon which he makes up his verdict. When the strong symptoms are all gathered together the physician in studying the case must separate out those things that were observed years ago from those things that are observed today, noting how they have changed and why changed. Sometimes they have been changed by drugs so that the whole nature of the economy is giving out a different group of symptoms.

The physician must learn the changes all along the line, from beginning to end; what symptoms represented this sick man ten years ago, and what symptoms represent him now. Perhaps now he has morbid anatomy, pathological conditions in his lungs, liver and kidneys. The physician who has been for twenty years observing previous and present conditions in this manner, by hearing the symptoms can practically locate the morbid anatomy; he can tell where it will appear, knows when pus is in organs and where, and he can fortell pretty well what is soon to go on in the economy. I would rather trust to a careful study of the symptoms than most physician's written diagnosis of phthisis, or organic diseases of the liver or of the heart. The symptoms do not lie, they do not exist from opinions of men who have thumped and pounded over the human body to find out what is going on inside, which is in many instances confusing even to the best diagnosticians. A considerable observation amongst medical men will lead one to discover that the dollar is the chief end of the practice of medicine when prac ticed in the old way; there is nothing else in it, nothing to admire or cherish.

To become conversant with symptoms, to judge of the sphere and progress of disease by the study of symptomatology, is the requirement necessary for the homœopath. Of course, bystanders will say to the patient, "That doctor cannot know much; he did not give you a physical examination." After the examination of the symptoms has been made there is no reason why you should not make a physical examination of the patient; but do not let this deprive you of becoming thoroughly educated in studying symptoms, because the real study of sickness is the meditation of his symptoms, and to become wise in symptoms is to become an able prescriber. Study physical diagnosis to your heart's content, but weigh carefully what you discover and compare it with the symptoms in order to ascertain what the different symptoms mean. You cannot study the symptoms of man without becoming extremely well acquainted with the nervous system. The anatomy of the nerves and of the brain should be thoroughly known. Not always that you may name the nerve, but that you may know where it is and what its functions are, and this study should be continued throughout all your life. The physician should be conversant with anatomy and physiology, but by studying the symptomatology he acquires a knowledge of physiology which it is impossible to obtain in any other way; he acquires a knowledge of the functions and operations of arteries, nerves and muscles because they call attention to themselves when in disturbance, and he sees therefore how the symptoms manifest themselves. By studying the symptom in the recorded pathogenesis one may learn much about true pathology. Morbid anatomy furnishes no basis for prescribing, but true pathology is often of the greatest benefit, helping the image of the sickness to shape itself before the mind.

LECTURE X

Several paragraphs now to be read are scarcely more than a recapitulation of subjects spoken of. In going over previous paragraphs I have introduced these points in advance, because it was natural to do so in connection with the subject in hand. I will therefore glance over them until we reach something new.

"In the thirteenth paragraph Hahnemann says:

"Therefore disease (that does not come within the province of manual surgery), considered, as it is by the allopathists, as a thing separate from the living whole, from the organism and its animating vital force, and hidden in the interior, be it of ever so subtle a character, is an absurdity that could only be imagined by minds of a materialistic stamp, and has for thousands of years given to the prevailing system of medicine all those pernicious impulses that have made it a truly mischievous (non-healing) art.

The material notion referred to was that existing in the time of Hahnemann Materialism is still growing. It seems impossible for the majority of men of the present day to perceive. Perception, that is, seeing with the understanding, seems to be entirely lost. The materialist refuses to believe anything that does not conform to the laws of time and space. It must be measured, it must be weighed, it must occupy space, or he has no idea of it, and will distinctly affirm that without this it is nothing and has no existence. Everything beyond this is to the material mind poetical, dreamy, mysterious. So they look in vain in the material world for cause. You will never find a material entity as in any way causing anything. It has no causative power, no creative influence, no propelling influence. Causes or simple substances are, in the natural state, in motion, and cause motion in the bodies that they occupy; the natural state for simple substance is that of power, of mobility, of activity. The natural state of matter is rest, quietude, silence; it has no power to move unless acted upon. Like the dead man, whose tissues are at rest, it has no action of its own. But the simple substance dominates matter and animates. it.

The two worlds, the world of motion, of power, and the world of inertia, exist in one. There is a world of life and a world of dead matter. The realm of thought and the realm of matter are the realm of cause and the realm of result. Causes are invisible, results are visible. We see the actions of material substance, but the thinking man has only to reflect to see that these actions that are visible in material form are but result of the cause that exist in the form of simple substance which is invisible to the natural eye but visible to the spiritual eye or understanding. The materialist cannot grasp this idea, he cannnot think in this way. We have the grandest confirmation of these things in the wonderful action of our potencies in the varying degrees in which they operate upon man, from the lowest to the highest. You will discover in course of time that in a large number of chronic diseases our antipsorics will cause changes in the economy, curative or otherwise, in from five to seven different potencies. In this you have the demonstration of degree of simple substance, and their relation to different planes in the interior of the economy.

§ 14. There is, in the interior of man, nothing morbid that is curable, and no invisible morbid alteration that is curable, which does not make itself known to the accurately observing physician by means of morbid signs and symptoms—an arrangement in perfect conformity with the infinite goodness of the all-wise Preserver of human life.

This we have already spoken of. Every curable disease is made known to the physician by signs and symptoms. Incurable diseases have few signs and symptoms, and by their absence the disease is often thus known to be incurable. By watching the patient gradually decline without any symptoms but those which are the common expressions of pathological conditions, we see that the case is incurable and is going down to death.

All curable maladies, therefore, have signs and symptoms in order to make themselves known; their purpose is to shadow forth the disorderly condition of the vital force or interior of man, so that the physician may read it and understand its nature. This imaging forth when the human race is in a state of ignorance, or materialism, is like seeds sown upon stony ground; there is no man to understand them, to apprehend their meaning. The images of sickness are continually being formed, and only wait for a man intelligent enough to observe them, to understand their meaning to translate them, and it is possible for men, by the doctrines of

Homœopathy, to become wise and intelligent enough to be conversant with these signs.

In this paragraph we also see Hahnemann's recognition of Divine Providence. It was the very recognition of Providence that enabled Hahnemann to become a man, and being directed by Divine Providence enabled him to finally perccive the law. When his little ones were being hurled to death by strong drugs the first thought of Hahnemann was that Providence had not made these little ones to be destroyed by medioino; it sccmcd to him inconsistent that they should be made to take this miserable stuff. In all your experiences, if you live to be very old, you will find a very poor lot of homœopaths among those who do not recognize Divine Order. You will find among them false science, experimentation, but never any government of principle, no thought of purpose, order or use.

Hahnemann was not in the strictest sense the discoverer of the law, for Hippocrates said that disease might be caused either by opposites or similars, but Hahnemann discovcred this by pure experimentation and the following out of strict order. After reading it up he found corroboration of the principles he had discovered, and he followed along the line, growing wiser and stronger, until he formulated tho codc which is so simple and yet so complete. Very few are able to read the *Organon* at first and see anything in it but words, and yet the oldest practitioner of pure Homœopathy finds nothing in it to change and the older he grows and becomes more active in work the more he depends upon it and the more consistent it becomes. Although I have been teaching the *Organon* for many years, I never go over it without discovering some new thought in harmony with the general teaching. The continued study of the *Organon* brings a deeper and deeper understanding of it, because it is true.

In the 15th paragraph another thought comes up which still further shows the unit of government which we have dwelt upon so much in past lectures. Everything that flows from a center must be considered in connection with that center. Man in his healthy state is but the result of the normal activities of a unit, and he must be considered as a unit. In other words, his healthy vital force is the result of action from a Center. On the otherhand, when man becomes diseased in his disordered or' diseased state he is still a unit and has to be considered collectively. It is not to be considered that his physiological action produces his morbid actions, but that his morbid actions so completely dominate him that he is one morbid state. This is again illustrated when he is dominated by the action of a drug (when a drug instead of a disease possesses him), then we see a morbid state, but it is still a unit of action.

There are three different subjects forming a union of study, the study of man in his natural state, the study of man in his sick state from natural disorder, and the study of man in his sick state from artificial disorder. Each remedy must be studied as a unit first and then those units may be compared. To intermingle comparative Materia Medica without a full knowledge of units is a mistake. This I have found out by experience in my earlier teaching. I have taught much comparative Materia Medica, thinking that a wise course to pursue, but have since abandoned that plan and now study each remedy as a unit, just as I advise the study of each disease as a unit. When one remedy is fully mastered, or one disease is fully mastered, then you are ready to compare. First of all think of measles as measles, and whooping cough as whooping cough, and, when you come to the chronic diseases, ascertain all the things that have been observed in syphilis, and all the symptoms that have been observed in sycosis, and all those that have been observed in psora. You are then prepared to enter the study of the Materia Medica and see the relationship of some remedies to the acute miasms and the relationship of other remedies to the chronic miasms. You will see particularly the image of measles in some remedies, the image of whooping cough in others, and the image of psora, syphilis and sycosis in others. Then you are ready to proceed with what may be called individualization, because these are the most general, and from these we go into particulars and then into comparison. This is the classical way to proceed, and when it is followed the physician becomes wise and intelligent and can apply the Materia Medica with wonderful precision. Such was Hahnemann's method.

LECTURE XI

§ 16. (1) Healthy State. (2) How made Sick. (3) How Cured.
Only Deranged and Cured in Dynamic Planes

Organon § 16. Our vital force, as a spirit-like dynamis, cannot be attacked
and infected by injurious influences on the healthy organism caused by the
external inimical forces that disturb the harmonious play of life otherwise
than in a spirit-like (dynamic) way, and in like manner all such morbid
derangements (diseases) cannot be removed from it by the physician in any
other way than by the spirit-like (dynamic, virtual), alternative powers of the
serviceable medicines acting upon our spirit-like vital force, which perserves
them through the medium of the sentient faculty of the nerves everywhere
present in the organism, so that it is only by their dynamic action of the
vital force that remedies are able to re-establish and do actually re-establish
health and vital harmony *after* the changes in the health of the patient cognizable by our senses (the totality of the symptoms) have revealed the disease
to the carefully observing and investigating physician as fully as was requisite
in order to enable him to cure it.

The 16th paragraph furnishes the subject that we will talk about
this morning. It treats of three states: (1) of the state of health,
or the normal activities of the body, (2) of how that state is made
sick or turned into disorder, and (3) of how that disordered state
can be turned into health. If we could find a man in a state of perfect health, we might subject him to shock, to injuries, to the
actions of the cruder things around us, and he would pass through
them or they would pass away without leaving upon him any such
thing as a disorder. He might be under the influence of that shock
a short time, but when reaction came, if it came at all, it would
leave him free from miasm, he would not have therefrom either an
acute or chronic disease. It is only by the action of immaterial substances, simple substances acting upon a plane similar to the plane
of his susceptibility, that he can become infected with a sickness;
that is, the resultant action of a substance capable of operating
from his innermost to his outermost, and establishing evidence
which we call symptoms. If the outermost alone is acted upon the
vital force of the man is only temporarily disturbed, but there is
not established a definite disorder (not even a limited one) that
can run a course with a beginning, a period of progress and decline,
such as the miasms do.

Whatever depresses the tissues of man, or his bodily functions, only acts temporarily, and is not capable of establishing a true disease. Take, for instance, the cruder drugs that we see used as a physic. You may give the patient the coarser and cruder forms of drugs as purgatives and emetics, and he will go through the shock and return to his original state. It is only after the most violent and long continued use of liquids that there can be implanted upon him a drug disease, and even that is largely superficial in comparison to a natural diseased condition. The constant use of Bromide of Potassium will produce effects in time, but that drug does not go to the depths, it operates upon the tissues, producing a coarser form of disease, but not miasmatic in character. Take also the coarser poisons as an example. Many of them can be taken into the stomach in crude form with very little manifestation upon the vital force, indeed the more active and virulent and condensed the poison the smaller the collective symptoms image. The smallpox crust can be swallowed and it will be digested and very little trouble come from it, but the inhalation of the atmosphere that contains the aura of smallpox upon a plane corresponding to the susceptibility of the individual will bring him down with the disease having a definite prodrome, a period of progress and a period of decline, showing that the very foundation of the man's nature has been struck. Such an operation is upon the internals of man upon his invisible, immaterial substance, and it operates from within out, producing ultimates in his tissues, establishing results upon the skin.

Hahnemann in this paragraph affirms that nothing, except in the form of a simple substance, can so implant itself upon the economy as to run its course as a disease either acute or chronic. No disease can implant itself upon the economy through its ultimate forms; only in its invisible forms can it so act. All diseases known to man are in the form of simple substance, an invisible something that cannot be detected by the chemist or the microscopist, and will never be detected in the natural world. Disease cause is known, and known only, from its effects; it is not capable of·investigation by the natural senses and can only be investigated as to its results. Everything that can be seen, felt or observed, or detected with the microscope, is but an ultimate , a result. It is only by the understanding, by reasoning from first to last and then back again, that we can perceive that disease causes are invisible.

The body can be affected, the tissues can be affected, and ulti-mates can be affected by ultimates, there can be friction between ultimates; things in this world can collide with other things in this world and they may destroy each other; ultimates may destroy ultimates; but such a thing as disease occurring in ultimates except through dynamic changes is impossible.

Nor can any agency which is an ultimate act upon the human economy curatively, turning into vital order the innermost of *life*. Vital disorder cannot be turned into order except by something similar in quality to the vital force. It is not similitude in quantity that we want, in weights and measures, but it is similarity in quality, in power, in plane, that must be sought for.

Medicines, therefore, cannot affect the high and interior planes of the physical economy unless they are raised to the plane of similarity in quality. The individual who needs Sulphur in the very highest degrees may take Sulphur sufficient to move his bowels, may rub it upon the skin, may wear it in his stockings, can take Sulphur baths, all without effect upon his disease. In that form the drug is not in correspondence with his sickness. it does not affect him in the same plane in which he is sick, and so it cannot affect the cause and flow from thence to the circumference. So with all the coarser drugs, they do not cure. We sometimes see the outer most effects of disease, disease located in the outer planes, tem-porarily removed by the lower potencies and crude drugs, but it is only as to the exteriors and ultimates that the cure is effected, and as it does not reach the innermost degrees it is not permanent. In acute diseases also crude drugs sometimes accomplish their pur-pose, because the outermost which they affect is only on the sur-face and the innermost has, in acute disease, the tendency to go away of itself; if his life can simply be spared until the disease has run its course the patient will recover. But the chronic miasms are only reached as to their ultimate symptoms, and these are caused to subside only temporarily or are suppressed by the action of the crude or ultimate forms of medicine.

I look back upon the time when my own mind was in a cloud as to this subject, and if I refer to it here it may be of use to you. I remember when I first read from Hahnemann that potentized medicines would cure the sick that it seemed to me a mystery. I had no knowledge upon which to found belief in such things. I began to practice with the lower potencies and with crude drugs in attempting to carry out the law, but with these means I was able to cure only superficial complaints. My work was far from satisfactory, yet it was somewhat better than the old things, it was milder than physicking and purging and emesis. Of course I rested upon my opinions and belief for my knowledge; everyone does that.

Later I resolved to test the 30th potency to see if there was not yet medicine in it, and I prepared with my own hands the 30th potency of Podophyllum with water on the centesimal scale, after the fashion of Hahnemann, having been told that water was as good as alcohol and it was only the attenuation that was required. This was during an epidemic of diarrhœa that looked like Podophyllum, but I had not the courage to give the 30th and still continued to use my stronger medicines. One day a child was brought into my office in the mother's arms. She brought it in hastily, and it did not seem as if it could live long. It was an infant, and while it lay in her arms a thin yellowish fecal stool ran over my carpet. The odor struck me as like that I had been reading about as the odor of the Podophyllum stool; it was horribly offensive, stinking, and the stool was so copious that the mother made the remark that she did not know where it all came from. I said to myself, this is a case upon which to test Hahnemann's 30th potency. So I fixed up some of the Podophyllum 30 and put it on the child's tongue, and sent the mother home, fearing that the child would soon die, as it was very ill, face pinched and drawn, cadaveric, and had a dreadful odor about it. Next morning when making my rounds I had to pass the house. I expected to see crepe on the door. I did not dare to call, though I was very much worried about it, so I drove past; but there was no crepe on the door. I drove home again that way, although it was quite a distance out of the way, and still there was no crepe on the door; but standing in the doorway was the grandmother, who said: "Doctor, the baby is all right this morning." Then I began to feel better, thinking I had not killed it. Perhaps some of you have been in the same state of mind.

That little child did not need any more medicine. After that I had quite a number of Podophyllum cases, and the 30th did the work to my astonishment. It was different from anything I had ever seen; the cures were almost instantaneous, it seemed as if there would be no more stool after the first dose of medicine. I did not always give the single dose. I used that 30th all the season, and then made up my mind that if the 30th of Podophyllum was good other 30ths would also be, and I ought to have as many of them as possible. I made a good many 30ths by hand, and finally succeeded in making up one hundred and twenty-six remedies, some of them in the 200th potency, and these I used. Then I procured a set of 200ths and higher and practiced with them. I followed on in this way and in a few years I discovered that by giving higher and higher potencies the remedies seemed to operate more and more interiorly,

I found that a chronic case that would be relieved by moderately high potencies would only improve for a matter of weeks, but on the administration of much higher potencies the work would be taken up, and in that way the same patient could be carried on from one potency to another. If I give you the conversation of one patient with me from time to time you may understand better what I mean. I saw this patient for the first time some fifteen years ago, when he was stoop-shouldered and had a fairly phthisical aspect. He had a catarrhal state of the chest, and it looked as though it might end in phthisis. On his symptoms he received Sulphur about 6 m. He was violently aggravated by this dose of medicine, all his symptoms were made worse, and he came back to the office saying that the medicine had made him sick. I had attained knowledge of the aggravation from a similar remedy, so I gave him sugar. At the end of another week he came back and told me he was better, much better, that he did not want me to give him any more of that first medicine, but he wanted more of the last, as it had made him so much better. So I kept him on the medicine which pleased him for a period of probably six or seven weeks. One time he returned and told me he did not want that last medicine, but he wanted that medicine that helped him so. By that I knew enough to give him another dose of Sulphur. Within the next day or two he ran in and said, "You young rascal, you gave me that medicine that made me sick in the first place," so he got sugar again and went on this time for five or six weeks, or perhaps longer. Then he came back again saying, "Now, I do not think you understand me, for I am having my old symptoms back. I wish you would study my case again." So I went all over his case and he got another dose of Sulphur 6 m. He reported this time, "Well, I do not feel any better; I am just about the same." He was not stirred up this time, you see. I waited a little longer and saw no relief from the last dose.

Here are all the symptoms calling for Sulphur, shall I give him crude Sulphur? I cannot give a remedy that is not indicated. The experience of the older men says "go higher." I gave him Sulphur 55 m., and in a few days he came back upon me, saying, "You rascal, you gave me that first medicine again. I don't want that stuff." Finally I got him cooled down, gave him some sugar and assured him that he would be better in a few days, and he went on for six or seven weeks with great improvement. After a while I explained to him that when the remedy did not act I had to give him something to stir him up. Of course I did not say anything to him about sugar.

When you have learned what your medicines will do it is a good thing to say to the patient, "Do not be alarmed or astonished when such and such things happen." Otherwise they will get alarmed and go off and perhaps get another doctor. The 55 m. of Sulphur relieved that patient in a couple of doses, far apart, and then ceased to relieve him any more. Next he received the c.m. which worked just as the other potencies had done, and finally he got to the mm. which acted just like the c.m., and from that poency he went on being restored to health. When you see these things you have a confirmation in them of the doctrines of the law. Experience does not lead to these things, but principles which thereafter are confirmed by experience. When a patient has been carried up through a series of potencies he will often remain unaffected by that remedy in a lower realm of potency or in the crude, unless he is overwhelmingly dosed by it, and then he will be poisoned.

The third proposition in this paragraph is that medicines will not act curatively, or in a way to turn the body into order and turn off disease, unless potentized to correspond to the degrees in which the man is sick. Such as are sick in a middle plane are sick from that plane to the outermost. Such as are sick in the interior planes are sick throughout to the outermost. When the disorder is in the very depth of his physical nature then it is in the form of chronic disease; i.e., all there is of him is sick, and of such there is no tendency to recovery but a continued progress. Such is the order of psora, syphilis and sycosis.

The nutritive plane is entirely in the outermost, that is, in the tissues. Assimilation goes on in the tissues. It is simply in the realm of tissues and ultimates that crude drugs operate; they can only disturb ultimates, and the inharmonious condition is the inharmony of ultimates, the outermost plane. Of course, if the outermost of the physical is disturbed the whole economy suffers, and the body ceases to furnish a good instrument to be operated upon by the powers within; but a *true disease*, with periods of prodrome, progress and decline or continuance, cannot be implanted upon the economy except it be by a dynamic cause. And hence necessarily man cannot be cured except by drugs attenuated until they have become similar to the nature or quality of disease cause. Disease cause and the disease-curing drug must be similar in nature; unlike causes would not produce like effects. We can arrive at similar causes by studying the effects that are similar. When we examine into a case and find a certain group of symptoms and in the effects produced by a certain drug we see like symptoms, we have a right to presume that the quality or nature in both is similar. The causes must be similar if the effects are similar in nature and quality. When the physician goes to the bedside he asks himself, Do I know a remedy that has produced, upon a healthy man, symptoms like these? He must pass judgment upon the symptoms, he must be an artist in application and capable of discerning the finer shades of difference and similitude.

LECTURE XII

Organon § 17. Now, as in the cure effected by the removal of the whole of the perceptible signs and symptoms of the disease the internal alteration of the vital force to which the disease is due—consequently the whole of the disease—is at the same time removed, it follows that the physician has only to remove the whole of the symptoms in order, at the same time, to abrogate and annihilate the internal change, that is to say, the morbid derangement of the vital force—consequently the totality of the disease, *the disease itself*. But when the disease is annihilated the health is restored, and this is the highest, the sole aim of the physician who knows the true object of his mission, which consists not in learned-sounding prating but in giving aid to the sick.

The idea of this paragraph is that the removal of the totality of the symptoms is actually the removal of the cause. It may not be known that causes are continued into effects (*i.e.*, that causes continue in ultimates), but it is true that all ultimates to a great extent contain the cause of the beginnings. And since cause continues into ultimates and things in ultimates shadow forth cause, the removal of all the symptoms will lead any rational man to assume that the cause has been removed. This will lead you to see that if a large number of symptoms manifest themselves through a diseased ovary, and that ovary is removed, the cause of the symptoms has not been removed and will manifest through some other part of the body, perhaps the other ovary or some organ that is weak.

It is a serious matter to remove any organ through which disease is manifested. When there are two or more of these pathological conditions established upon the body and one is removed the other immediately becomes worse. For instance, if there is a structural change in the knee joint and the surgeon removes the knee, while there is a corresponding structural change in the kidneys or liver which he cannot remove, the latter immediately becomes worse and breaks down as soon as the knee joint is removed. In the same way we find in a tuberculous condition of the lungs that it may remain in a very quiet state so long as a fistula *in ano* keeps on discharging but the allopath comes along and closes that vent and immediately there is a cropping out of the disease by infiltration of the lungs and the patient comes to an early death. The results of diseases are necessary in many instances. Sometimes these results are tuberculous conditions, which are the ultimate outcome or effects from cause, and contain at times the seeds of beginnings of a similar kind. They are not themselves beginnings, yet they contain causes. Unless causes are removed from beginning to end the disease can reproduce itself. This includes the first proposition of Hahnemann as to the cure of disease, which means permanent removal of the totality of the symptoms, thus removing the cause and turning disorder into order, and as a consequence the results of disease are removed. The totality cannot be removed without removing the cause.

"But when the disease is annihilated the health is restored; and this is the highest, the sole aim of the physician who knows the true object of his mission, which consists not in learned-sounding prating but in giving aid to the sick." Hahnemann gives this warning note against discoursing dogmatically upon the flimsy theories of man. It was the custom in Hahnemann's time for men to cloak their ignorance in technicalities; that is, to use technicalities for the purpose of appearing wise. It is done at the present day, I have heard physicians talk to simple-minded people in technicalities. Wise people seldom use technicalities. There is nothing in this world to becloud the understanding as to deal in technicalities, they are cramped and often meaningless. The doctrines of Homœopathy should not be clouded in technicalities, but should be considered and talked out in the simplest forms of speech. When talking of the *Organon* and its doctrines, talk good English, if you are English, and use simple forms of speech. One technical word will sometimes mean a whole sentence, and can be consistuted to mean a good many different things. Technicalities are a sort of scapegoat to carry off the sins of our ignorance.

The "totality of the symptoms" means a good deal. It is a wonderfully broad thing. It may be considered to be all that is essential of the disease. It is all that is visible and represents the disease in the natural world to the eye, the touch and external understanding of man. It is all that enables the physician to individualize between diseases and between remedies; the entire representation of a disease is the totality of the symptoms, and the entire representation of a drug is the totality of the symptoms. It does not mean the little independent symptoms, but it means that which will bring to the mind a clear idea of the nature of the sickness. Many of the little symptoms that occur can be left out of the total without marring, but the essence, the characteristics, the image must be there, as that is of importance to the physician, being to him the sole indication in the choice of the remedy. It is true that the old prescriber may be able to perceive the totality if he can see only a small portion of it. Prescribing in that way, however, is very often a mistake, for when that which was wanting is brought out the physician sees that he has prescribed only for the side view, as it were. You become well acquainted with old friends and know them by even a partial view or by the gait, or voice, but it is not so with strangers. Strangers have to be studied, criticized and examined. It requires a long time to know the stranger's methods, to find out how he performs his business, whether he is cheerful or not to know the character, to know the man. So it is with the totality of the symptoms, for to a great extent every sickness is a new sickness. If the patient has nothing to conceal he will delineate his symptoms cheerfully, but if he has something to conceal it becomes a hard matter to obtain the totality of his symptoms. But this totality must be obtained, for there is no other means of ascertaining the nature of the remedy that he is in need of, as it is expressed in the eighteenth paragraph:

From this indubitable truth, that, besides the totality of the symptoms, nothing can by any means be discovered in diseases wherewith they could express their need of aid, it follows undeniably that the sum of all the symptoms in each individual case of disease must be the *sole indication*, the sole guide to direct us in the choice of a remedy.

But it is not enough to consider the totality as a grand whole; besides considering all the symptoms collectively each individual symptom must be considered. Every symptom must be examined to see what relation it sustains to and what position it fills in that totality in order that we may know its value, whether it is a common symptom, whether it is a particular symptom, or whether a peculiarly characteristic symptom. This we shall consider later in the course.

§ 19. Now, as *diseases* are nothing more than *alterations in the state of health of the healthy individual* which express themselves by morbid signs, and the *cure* is only possible by a *change to the healthy condition of the state of health of the diseased individual,* it is very evident that *medicines* could never cure diseases if they did not possess the power of altering man's state of health, which depends on sensations and functions; indeed that their curative power must be owing *solely* to this power they possess of altering man's state of health.

The statement is that medicines must be capable of effecting changes in the economy or they cannot restore order in the economy. If the medicine is too high to effect a disturbance in an irregularly governed economy it will be too high to effect a cure in that economy. The potency must be consistent with the degree of susceptibility that calls for the medicine. This susceptibility includes a wide range of potency, so that from the 30th to the cm. there is seldom a miss in actual experience. It is seldom that the potency is too high, but that it is higher than is necessary is often true. No drug can act curatively except by its ability to effect changes, and it is known that drugs do effect changes by their provings; but in the provings the drug has been increased in quantity or reduced in quality in accordance with the judgment of the prover. Many times the coarser substances effect few changes and sometimes none, whereas the higher substances make sick; this is in accordance with the state of susceptibility. Some provers are susceptible to the higher who are not at all susceptible to the lower. There are patients who are not in the least susceptible to a single drop of tincture of Coffea but who are extremely susceptible to the higher potencies of Coffea. Such patients, however, are often made sick by large quantities of coffee. Lycopodium in its crude form has upon most people no effect, but in the higher potencies is capable, if followed up continuously, of affecting almost everyone. The effect that medicines have upon the sick in restoring order can best be observed by inducing the effects upon healthy individuals, which we call *proving.*

You might easily suppose, by the way the modern firms bring their medicines before us, that they have by a great effort of their will, and by great meditation, thought out what these drugs will do to the human family. For the purpose of ascertaining the state of medicine at the present time I very often listen patiently to a drummer from some of the New York houses. He will speak his piece, tell what this wonderful combination will do, how many diseases it will cure, and then I ask him how he finds this out.

"Oh, the doctors say so. Here are the testimonials." "But how do they find it out?" "Oh, they use them."

But the drugs have not been proved, and their use is not in accordance with what the homœopath knows the drugs will produce or cure. If you go into a friendly drug store and talk with the druggist you will find these medicines which have been concocted in the prescriptions of all the fashionable doctors in the neighbourhood. In six months from that time if you go to that same store you will not find one of those drugs in use, but a new set following the visit of the travelling man who has come around to represent their wonderful properties. Do not think that I refer entirely to the old school, because a large percentage of these prescriptions is from professed homœopaths, and that is as much Homœopathy as anything they do. The majority of homœopaths do these things, attempting to establish a homœopathic practice upon an allopathic foundation. They try to become fashionable and change their prescriptions as the ladies change their bonnets with the season.

In § 20 Hahnemann says:

This spirit-like power to alter man's state of health (and hence to cure diseases) which lies hidden in the inner nature of medicines can never be discovered by us by a mere effort of reason; it is only by experience of the phenomena it displays when acting in the state of health of man that we can become clearly cognizant of it.

There is only one way of finding out what Aconite will do to the economy, and that is to give it to many men and note the symptoms that these men experience as the manifestations of Aconite. It is first necessary to know that drugs can make man sick, and next to know what that state of sickness is. Every medicine that a homœopath uses should have been thoroughly proven upon the healthy so that its symptom image shall have been thoroughly brought out. It is a burning shame upon the homœopathic profession that so large a number of drugs exist in the homœopathic pharmacies, and that these drugs are recommended for such and such diseases without any investigation as to their properties, other than perhaps that Dr. So-and-So, on the recommendation of some old woman, has used this or that drug for dropsy. Such a thing is positively condemned in every line of the *Organon* and by every doctrine. There is no principle in it, it is unscientific, and unworthy of the vocation of a doctor. Every drug must be thoroughly proven upon the healthy. In our study of the Materia Medica I do not encumber you with partially proved drugs. We can study these after we have studied those that have been well proved. The "Guiding Symptoms" contain many medicines only partially proven, and it is often a matter of accident when cures are made with them. But the old remedies that have been handed down from the masters, and that have had years of trial, come to us as friends which we can learn of and become acquainted with. You cannot become acquainted with unproved drugs. When books tell you that a drug is good for this or that pay no attention to them, but when a book tells you that a drug has produced such and such symptoms study these; that is a piece of valuable information. The old school Materia Medica is made up of the results of medicine upon sickness, an unscientific guide, a fluctuating scale.

LECTURE XIII

THE LAW OF SIMILARS

[READ ORGANON § 21-25.]

In these paragraphs Hahnemann summarizes what he has said before and points out the necessary conclusions. In doing so he proves that the only method of applying medicines profitably in disease is the homœopathic method. We daily see that the anti-pathic and heteropathic methods have no tendency of permanency in their results. By these means there are effected changes in the economy and changes in the symptoms but no permanent cure, the tendency being simply to the establishment of another disease, often worse than the first, and without eradicating the first. In this connection we might speak of the giving of morphine and purgatives. The friends of the patient plead with you to stop the pain or give something to move the bowels for the relief of the patient. You know quite well that the relief from morphine is very transient, but when you are occupying the ground of principle there is the strongest reason why a dose of morphine should never be administered. After giving morphine changes are observed which are really detrimental to the patient. The symptoms are changed, and this is always unfortunate. The same objection applies to the giving of chloroform in labor. No woman at the present day is well enough to go through labor without some symptoms calling for a remedy. Hence, if you give chloroform in labor, you put your patient in a state in which she is unable to express the symptoms of her own condition. If, at the close of labor, she was about to give forth symptoms that would indicate to the intelligent physician what remedy she needed (perhaps to overcome a life-time of suffering) you would be deprived of knowing what the remedy was by this act of foolishness.

§ 26. This depends on the following homœopathic law of nature which was sometimes, indeed, vaguely surmised but not hitherto fully recognized, and to what is due every real cure that has ever taken place:

A weaker dynamic affection is permanently extinguished in the living organism by a stronger one, if the latter (whilst differing in kind) is very similar to the former in its manifestation.

In this paragraph Hahnemann distinctly declares that the phenomena of cure depend entirely upon fixed law, the law of similars or the law that governs Homœopathy. After Hahnemann had made a number of provings he gathered together from the literature a great number of reported cures for the purpose of observing whether the cures had been made accidentally or from purpose and whether they were in accordance with the law of similars or with the principle of dissimilars. In every instance he was able to see that the cures had been made in accordance with the law of similars, viz., that the drug which cured in each case was capable of producing symptoms similar to those which it cured. This is true in all planes, under all circumstances, and all other apparent cures are not cures but suppressions.

"A dynamic disease in the living economy of man is extinguished in a permanent manner by another that is more powerful when the latter (without being of the same species) bears a strong resemblance to it in its mode of manifesting itself." That sentence seemed to be about the best way of expressing the law in Hahnemann's time. The words "more powerful," or more intense, would afford a natural way of expressing it, but when one has lived in Homœopathy, and has been able to perceive its inner workings, the word "powerful" expresses a different thought. If we follow along the line of potentization we lose the idea of power that is manifest to an uninitiated mind. We enter the world of thought and therein learn of a different kind of power or intensity. When we think naturally of power or intensity the mind is at once carried to the idea of intensity as in an electrical problem in which we increase the intensity by increasing the number of batteries. On the other hand, Hahnemann's expression leads to the idea of intensity, having qualities more internal, higher, prior; i.e., in the sense of from first to last, the more internal it is the more intense, the more it approaches the first substance, so that intensity as to cause means higher or more internal, higher in the sense of subtleness or fineness.

The word "powerful" then, you will please note, contains an interior thought, and that is the only way to bring the mind to realize what is meant. Powerful is actually from within and hence we potentize, going higher and higher, in order that we may reach intensity, and it is in this sense that the remedy becomes more powerful by potentization. As a matter of fact, when speaking

upon the material plane, the remedy grows weaker by potentization because the material is actually reduced. It would seem strange
to a materialist, to an old school doctor for instance, who has not
thought of anything but the giving of great pills, to say that
Aconite becomes more powerful by being attenuated. To him it
would just be saying that it becomes more powerful the weaker it
becomes and yet it is really so, though he cannot see it.

"A dynamic disease is extinguished by another that is more
powerful when the latter is similar to it." The first proposition is
that it must be similar and then it must be intense enough. The
more there is in the interior, the more there to expect in the
exterior. So it is with the light of the sun. It is grander than all
other lights, because there is more in its interior; it is purer, it is
more dynamical and it will turn aside and destroy all other light.

This law of similars is seen prominently in the natural world. We
see it from man to man. It is easily illustrated among the insane. It
is the secret of mind cure, and there are many instances of mind
cure that are based on the law of similars. One example of this is
seen in the young girl who has lost her mother or lover and is ill
as a consequence, is depressed with grief, is constantly sobbing,
and has become melancholy. She sits in a corner, hears nobody,
thinks no one can pity her because no one has had just such grief.
Let us apply allopathic treatment to her. "Come, there is nothing
the matter with you; why don't you brace yourself up; why don't
you try to arouse yourself?" But this only throws her into a deeper
state of melancholy. Scolding and harsh treatment do no good.
But introduce the homœopathic treatment, employ a nurse if you
will who is a good actress and who has gone through the same
identical grief, and let her make a big fuss in the other corner.
Pretty soon the patient will say, "You seem to have the same grief
that I have." "Yes, I have lost a lover." "Well, you can sympathize
with me," and the two fall to bellowing and weep it out together.
There is a bond of sympathy. Sometimes a curable case of insanity
can be reached in this way, and thus we have a mind cure. Hahnemann made use of this plan in curing insanity. When a patient
would exert her will, but is unable on account of the physical
encumbrances, then the homœopathic remedy will restore order.

§ 27. The curative power of medicines, therefore depends on their symptoms, similar to the disease but superior to it in strength, so that each
individual case of disease is most surely, radically, rapidly and permanently

annihilated and removed only by a medicine capable of producing (in the human system) in the most similar and complete manner the totality of its symptoms, which at the same time are stronger than the disease.

Then it is not sufficient merely to give the drug itself regardless of its form. It is not sufficient to give the crude drug, but the plane upon which it is to be given is a question of study. The attenuation also must be similar to the disease cause. In a proving the crude drug may bring forth a mass of symptoms in one prover, but when a person is sick those symptoms will not be touched by the crude drug because the patient does not sustain the similar relation or susceptibility that the one did who proved it.

In paragraph 29, Hahnemann has given an explanation of the law of cure. He himself preludes it by saying that he does not attach much importance to it. You are not in any way bound to consider it, and it is usually omitted in this course.

LECTURE XIV

SUSCEPTIBILITY

Oraganon § 30

The human body appears to admit of being much more powerfully affected in its health by medicines (partly because we have the regulation of the dose in our own power) than by natural morbid stimuli—for natural diseases are cured and overcome by suitable medicines.

§ 31. The inimical forces, partly psychical, partly physical, to which our terrestrial existence is exposed, which are termed morbific noxious agents, do not possess the power of morbidly deranging the health of man unconditionally; but we are made ill by them only when our organism is sufficiently disposed and susceptible to the attack of the morbific cause that may be present and to be altered in its health, deranged and made to undergo abnormal sensations and functions, hence they do not produce disease in everyone, nor at all times.

§ 32. But it is quite otherwise with the artificial morbific agents which we term medicines. Every real medicine, namely, acts at *all* times, under *all* circumstances, on *every* living human being, and produces in him its peculiar symptoms (distinctly perceptible if the dose be large enough) so that evidently every human organism is liable to be affected, and, as it were, inoculated with the medical disease, at all times and absolutely (unconditionally), which, as before said, is by no means the case with the natural disease.

Incidentally these paragraphs have a bearing upon degree or intensity (which is potentization), upon the repetition of the dose, and upon susceptibility, things which must be known by the homœopathic physician in order that he may be a good prescriber. We have studied potentization sufficiently to see that disease causes exist among attenuated things, the infinitesimal or immaterial substances, and thus the physician must see that the curative remedy must be on the same plane. He must know why it is that he should give but one dose, and the rationale by which susceptibility is satisfied.

In contagion (and consequently in cure) there is practically but one dose administered, or at least that which is sufficient to cause a suspension of influx. When cause ceases to flow in a particular direction it is because resistance is offered for causes flow only in the direction of least resistance and so when resistance appears influx ceases, the cause no longer flows in. Now in the beginning of disease, *i.e.*, in the stage of contagion, there is this limit to influx, for if man continued to receive the cause of disease (if there were no limits to its influx) he would receive enough to kill him, for it would run a continuous course until death. But when susceptibility is satisfied, there is a cessation of cause, and when cause ceases to flow into ultimates, not only do the ultimates cease but cause itself has already ceased.

Hahnemann states that we have more power over human beings with durgs than disease cause, for man is only susceptible to natural diseases upon a certain plane. Disease causes, existing as they do as immaterial substances, flow into man in spite of him; he can neither control nor resist them, and they make him sick. But certain changes occur and man ceases to be susceptible, and there is no longer an inflowing of cause into his economy; a suspension has taken place, because susceptibility has ceased. Susceptibility ceases when changes occur in the economy that bar out any more influx.

But cure and contagion are very similar, and the principles applying to one apply to the other. There is this difference: in cure we have the advantages of change of potency, and this enables us to suit the varying susceptibilities of sick man. Because of these varying degrees of susceptibility some are protected from disease cause and some are made sick; the one who is made sick is susceptible to the disease cause in accordance with the plane he is in and the degree of attenuation that happens to be present at the time of contagion. The degree of the disease cause fits his susceptibility at the moment he is made sick. But it is not so with medicines. Man has all the degrees of potentization, and by these he can make changes and thereby fit the medicine to the varying susceptibility of man in varying qualities or degrees. Hence Hahnemann writes "Medicines (particularly as it depends on us to vary doses according to our will) appear to have greater power in affecting the state of health than the natural morbific irritation, for natural diseases are cured and subdued by appropriate medicines."

Now, here we might ask the question, when does a medicine that has been administered cease to be homœopathic? The same principle as to susceptibility must apply, because of the similarity between cure and contagion. Let me illustrate it in this way. Suppose we have a case of diphtheria, and after due study Lachesis appears to be the most similar of all medicines and a dose is given. Now, when does Lachesis cease to be homœopathic? When the symptoms that indicated it change, then it is no longer indicated. If it is given at all after this change, it operates upon a different plane from what it did in its homœopathicity, and if it acts at all it does not act curatively but depressingly. Any more than just enough to supply the susceptibility is a surplus and is dangerous. In a chronic disease administer Sulphur when it is clearly indicated, and the symptoms disappear and the patient feels better. Then the remedy ceases to be homœopathic, and if it is administered longer whatever action it has, is neither homœopathic nor desirable.

But man argues if a little will do good, more will do more good. Enough to effect a change is all that can be homœopathic; when certain changes are effected then the physician must wait.

Enough medicine must be given to establish order, and that is done almost instantaneously; at most it is but a matter of a few hours, and as long as order continues after it has once begun, so long "hands off." That is just the way contagion takes place. In diphtheria the disease begins, susceptibility ceases, a change takes place that protects the man from any further disease cause flowing into the body, and the disease develops and manifests itself by its symptoms.

The repetition of dose is advised by many wise heads, but if we understand this doctrine it will be clear to us that such repetition of dose is perfectly useless. It is true, that in vigorous, robust subjects who have lightning-like reaction the dose may be repeated and changes occur for the better if the remedy is not quite homœopathic to the case. But some are injured in this way because they are delicate subjects, whose reaction is slow; the reaction is actually prevented by the repetition of the dose; i.e., the order we have tried to establish is actually prevented. Hahnemann teaches that the human economy is more under control of man than under the control of disease, for the economy can be affected only by such disease as it is susceptible to, but man, whether for the purpose of proving or for the purpose of curing, can so vary the dose that he can always get results, and the very susceptible ones are terribly damaged by the repetition of the dose.

In the thirty-first paragraph Hahnemann says that disease causes are limited in their ability to effect changes in health, to certain conditions and states; *i.e.*, to susceptibility. This is all Hahnemann says of this doctrine of cessation of cause after certain evolutions have taken place. We see that when a natural disease is taken it runs its period, and tends to decline, and the patient will not be susceptible until another change of state has arrived. It is not true that man will go out of one state of susceptibility to a disease, and in a few days go into another state of susceptibility to that same disease. There must be a change, a cycle, which means a certain length of time. Now if we talk about cure instead of contagion, it would seem that a certain dose of medicine administered had lasted a certain time.

That is commonly the appearance. The medicine appears to act all that time, and you should be clear in your mind that this is only an appearance. It really means that a certain length of time elapses before another dose is necessary, viz., until another state of susceptibility has arrived. So again we say, whenever a medicine ceases to be homœopathic it is of no use to administer that medicine any longer, as it will act on the patient only upon an artificial susceptibility. By this we mean that certain sensitive patients always have a susceptibility to high potencies. We have thus two things to deal with, the actute state, created by the disease itself, and the chronic state, which is the natural state of the patient born under miasm. Now, when in the acute state the patient has satisfied the susceptibility to contagion, there is a period in which the disease cause can no longer operate upon him; he is immune against any further influx of disease cause. But when a remedy ceases to be homœopathic, the patient has not this immunity against more of its power because of the possibility of variance in the hands of the physician; the potency being given to the patient outside of his own degree of susceptibility, he may be damaged.

§ 33. In accordance with this fact it is undeniably shown by all experience that the living human organism is much more disposed and has a greater liability to be acted on and to have its health deranged by medicinal powers, than by morbific noxious agents and infectious miasms; or in other words, *that the morbific noxious agents possess a power of morbidity deranging man's health that is subordinate and conditional, often very conditional; whilst medicinal agents have an absolute unconditional power, greatly superior to the former.*

When we look over the improper use of all sorts of medicines, we can but conclude that the human race, because of drug-taking, has been greatly disordered in the economy. You have heard Hahnemann speak of the management of chronic diseases; he distinctly states that the greatest difficulties are those that have been brought about in the economy by continuous drug taking. It is not that the drugs themselves are laid up in the economy, but that life-long disorder is created. Think of the poor old individuals who were in the habit of taking sulphur and molasses, think of those who were perpetually tapping their livers with blue mass, think of the western sufferers who have filled themselves every year with quinine pan-cake to keep off the chill. These people are so disordered that it takes years of careful prescribing to turn them into a state of order.

In § 34 Hahnemann repeats two propositions to which we have already alluded. The first proposition is that in order to cure the medicines must be able to produce in the human body an artificial disease similar to that which is to be cured; this has been fully illustrated and explained. The second proposition is that the artificial disease must be of a greater degree of intensity. The matter of intensity has already been explained as something higher, more internal, something superior or prior. Intensity of power is proportionate to the degree of approximation towards primitive substance. There is no thought of intensity in any other direction. The cause of disease and of cure exists within the primitive substance and not in ultimate material form, although the immaterial cause of disease continues in disease ultimates. The bacteriologists have crawled into confusion because they do not know in their science that causes continue into effects. The bacteria may contain cause because causes are continued into ultimates; but the primitive cause is not in the bacteria; the bacteria themselves have a cause.

LECTURE XV

PROTECTION FROM SICKNESS

ORGANON § 35 *et seq.*

From these paragraphs we see that there are several kinds of protection from sickness. When a violent epidemic is raging we all know that, although the number of victims is large, they are few compared to those who go through the epidemic unscathed, and the question always arises, why is it? We suppose, and probably rightly so, that a large number of the immune have escaped because they were usually strong and vigorous, or in a state of very good order. But we find among those who have escaped the epidemic a number of persons who are anything but strong, really invalids, one in consumption, another in the last stages of Bright's disease, another with diabetes. We call them all together and find that none of them have had dysentery or smallpox, or whatever disease was epidemic. They have not been susceptible to epidemic influences. How are you going to explain this? The reason is that they have sickness that it is impossible for the epidemic to suppress. The epidemic is allopathic, or dissimilar to their diseases, and cannot suppress their disease because of its virulency. Now if they have some mild form of chronic disease, a severe attack of dysentery will cause that disease to disappear temporarily, and the new (epidemic) disease will take hold and run its course, and when it subsides the old symptoms will come back again and go on as if they had not been meddled with. This is an illustration of dissimilars, and shows that dissimilars are unable to cure: they can only suppress. If the chronic disease is stronger than the epidemic disease, *i.e.*, if it has an organic hold upon the body, it cannot be suppressed. This is essentially the relation of the acute dissimilar disease to the chronic disease of severity.

The relation between chronic dissimilar diseases is somewhat different. For example, a patient is in the earlier stages of Bright's disease, and the symptoms are clear enough to make a diagnosis. He takes syphilis, and at once the kidney disease is held in abeyance, the albumin disappears from the urine and his waxiness is

lost. But after a year's careful prescribing the syphilitic state disappears, and very soon the albumin appears again in the urine,
the dropsy returns and he dies of an ordinary attack of Bright's
disease.

Then there are cases where two chronic diseases seem at times
to alternate with each other; one seems to be subdued for a time
and the other prevails. Under proper homœopathic treatment one
will be reduced in its activity and the other chronic disease will
show itself. This you will find to be the case when you have to
treat syphilis and psora together. The psoric patient, who has been
suffering from a skin eruption or one of the various forms of psora,
takes syphilis. All the psoric manifestations, the nightly itching of
the salt rheum will disappear, and the syphilitic eruption will come
on and take their place. You will treat the syphilitic manifestations
for a while and you will be able to subdue them, and in proportion as the disease is subdued the psoric manifestations will come
up again and will hold in abeyance that portion of the syphilitic
state which is still uncured. You will then be compelled to drop
the anti-syphilitic and take up the anti-psoric treatment, and again
the homœopathic remedies will restore apparent order in the
economy. But after this has been done, you will be surprised to
see syphilitic state return in the condition corresponding to its last
manifestations. You must then drop the anti-psoric treatment and
resume the anti-syphilitic. Thus they alternate; when you weaken
one, the stronger comes up. The uncomplicated syphilitic eruption
does not itch; but the psoric eruption as a rule is an itching eruption, and this will be seen in the alternation of the two diseases.

If the patient is given proper treatment his condition will be
simplified, but if given old school treatment it will become very
complicated. The two miasms will unite and form a complexity,
which is a most vicious state of affairs; then the syphilitic eruptions,
while they have all the appearance of syphilis, will itch as if they
were psoric eruptions. Mercury in large doses is capable of bringing about such a result. Proper homœopathic treatment causes a
separation, while inappropriate treatment produces complication,
and you will never see one improve where homœopathic remedies
have caused the tying up of the combination.

Again, take a chronic malarial diathesis, which has existed so long
that it has complicated itself with psora, we will see after the
quinine has been antidoted that the chills and fever will come back

in their original form. Here you see an evidence of the separation which Homœopathy always tends to bring about. The malarial state is now brought into observation for the purpose of cure. It cannot be cured when complicated, for the remedy cannot be clear that will be similar enough to wipe them out. The first prescription antidotes the drug and liberates the patient from the drug disease, and then you see the most acute or last appearing natural disease which comes back first. This is in accordance with fixed law; the last miasm or the last symptoms that have been made to disappear will be the first to return and go away to appear no more.

In § 36 another thought comes up: "Thus non-homœopathic treatment, which is not violent, leaves the chronic disease unaltered. To suppress, there is required a state of violence to be brought about upon the body; one must do violence to the economy by enormous dosing, tremendous physic, much sweating, blood-letting, etc., such as was done in olden times. Such treatment tends to subdue or suppress disease for the time being; but when the violence has subsided and the rough treatment is removed then the symptoms come back, but in a more disturbed state than before. The more violent the drug disease that can be established upon the body the greater the changes in the chronic disease. Violent treatment alters the nature of the chronic diseases. A new and more intense disease suspends a prior dissimilar one existing in the body; similarly, just so long as the effect of quinine continues, so long will it suppress and hold in abeyance the disease to which it is dissimilar. Quinine is capable of engrafting upon the economy its own disease form which will last for years and may not stop until it has been antidoted by a medicine similar to its symptoms. But if it is antidoted, that malarial disease which it suppressed will appear in its original form and the patient will say: "These are just the symptoms I had in the first place when I was cured by the late Dr. So-and-so; he cured me with Peruvian bark." That story is so common that any homœopathic physician who has been doing sound prescribing for years has lots of records of just such cases. The malaria was subdued only because the quinine was capable of producing a more violent disease than malaria. Arsenicum is capable of doing the same thing; it can engraft upon the economy a dangerous disease that will result in very serious conditions because the Arsenicum will complicate itself with psora.

In some cases we have a complexity of horrible things, like one built upon another, and when this is so, in treating them the last group which was removed will appear first, which shows that the remedy has done its work, and we then go on to the next, and so on, the different groups sometimes appeared one after another in distant form. They must disappear in the reverse order of their coming, as if put on in layers, one piled upon another.

From all this we see how it is possible for two different diseases to occupy, as it were, two different corners of the same economy, one manifesting itself while the other is subdued. We also see how they may exist in a state of complexity. In the first instance they do not combine, in the other they do and become complex. We also see the propriety and use of observing what treatment has been administered to the patient. It is not always possible to do this, and it is impossible to know whether each one of these drugs has established its own disease.

Not every drug that is administered is capable of establishing a disease. It is always prudent, when symptoms are only partially developed, and when the drug which caused the suppression of symptoms is known, to include the antidotal relation to the drug with the rest of the symptoms; that is to say, select a drug which has a well-known antidotal relation to the drug that caused the suppression of the symptoms, providing it is also the most similar of all drugs to the few symptoms that are present. In that way we make as much of similitude as is possible. The similar remedy is most likely of all others to antidote that drug. Do not be led aside to administer right away the drug that caused the trouble. The principle of *Similia* is first.

43. Totally different, however, is the result when *two similar* diseases meet together in the organism; that is to say, when to the disease already present a stronger similar one is added. In such cases we see how a cure can be effected by the operations of nature, and we get a lesson as to how man ought to cure.

Then a real conjunction takes place, a union, as it were, a marriage, which results in the disappearance of old things and new things come and exist in a state of order.

LECTURE XVI

OVERSENSITIVE PATIENTS

ORGANON § 44 et seq.

Drug poisoning such as we referred to in last lecture is not always due to the prescribing of crude drugs. If you work long among sensitive patients you will come across those who have been actually poisoned by the inappropriate administration of potentized medicines. These are oversensitive patients who have received repeated doses of medicine after the medicine and dose that was homœopathic to their condition was administered.

If a drug that is really homœopathic to the case is continued, after enough has been given to cure, a miasm is established in some cases by that drug, and this miasm imitates one of the chronic diseases or one of the acute miasms in accordance with its ability. I have a patient who has been suffering for seven or eight years from the effects of Lachesis. I have patients who are suffering from Sulphur and other deep acting medicines which have been repeated too often when truly indicated, or repeated in sensitive patients when not truly indicated. The symptoms of the drug crop out periodically years after it has been abused, and the periodical attacks are perfectly typical of the drug. The mineral substances which are perfectly harmless on the crude plane may be poisonous on the dynamic plane, when the patient is oversensitive. There are persons who can drink a glass of milk with impunity and be nourished by it, but upon whom a drop of milk, potentized to a high degree and repeated beyond its homœopathicity, will establish a miasm that will last for years. A prover of Lac-caninum had a return of its symptoms periodically. She was an oversensitive and proved the medicine indiscriminately, and has suffered ever since from its poisonous effects, whereas if it had been given prudently, the disease would have established itself upon the body like any other acute miasm, would have run its course and disappeared. It is unwise to make provings upon oversensitive subjects in that way. I tested a very high potency of Lachesis on an oversensitive patient, giving but a single dose, and that patient ran the course of the Lachesis disease in about two months; the symptoms disappeared and never returned. While the Lachesis was in progress the patient's chronic symptoms were suppressed, but after it ran its course and disappeared her chronic symptoms came back. This is in accordance with the doctrines. She was oversensitive, and while the dissimilar Lachesis disease was in full blast her chronic disease was suppressed. These are instances when such a patient is truly homœopathic to a remedy, and if that remedy be repeated after enough (I mean in the internal sense) has been given to cure it ceases its homœopathic relation and acting through the general susceptibility creates a miasm upon this extremely sensitive patient. When a patient is hypersensitive you must avoid the use of the c.m. and other very high potencies, which will make your patient sick, and use instead the 30th and 200ths. In cases where the remedy is indicated such potencies will work quite quickly.

§ 49. We should have been able to meet with many more real natural homœopathic cures of this kind, if, on the one hand, the attention of observers had been more directed to them and, on the other hand, if nature had not been so deficient in helpful homœopathic diseases.

Hahnemann, in § 46, gives examples of these natural cures. We occasionally meet with these cures now. We find patients that are threatened with phthisis go to the South, because it has been proved that such cases can go into a vitiated climate and stay for a number of years, and actually receive benefit from this disease-producing neighbourhood, and go away well. Others go into a climate more wholesome and they are not cured. The miasms can cure all similar diseases, and the curing substances are in attenuated form. The evils that arise from these swamps are similar to the evils of the economy of the patient, and that similitude is antidotal, is curative, and causes change back into order in accordance with the eternal law that governs the action of similars.

There was a time in the early days of Homœopathy when, taking into view the great array of disease forms to be contended with and the very few medicines then at his command, the homœopath was worried to find remedies similar to all of his cases. That cannot be true now. If the homœopath will work in a systematic way, he will be able to command enough of the Material Medica to meet all the diseases that he comes in contact with, the symptoms of which are sufficiently observed.

Every man should put himself to the task of studying the Materia Medica; he has no time to lose, no time to fool away. The physician can really have no excuse at the present day to leave our proved medicines, the medicines that are recorded in our books; he can have no reasonable excuse for stepping aside into ways that are dark, treacherous and recommended only by tradition. Some physicians hold that it is liberal to do anything for a patient. This is a pitfall, a rock, that will destroy any physician that will not avoid it. We know that there are doctors, who claim to be homœopaths, who attempt to justify, upon some ground or other, the administration of remedies merely to palliate and relieve suffering. With such men there must be a lack of sturdiness in listening to the sufferings of a patient. It seems to me that no one who is honest, and who has knowledge of the stupidity that comes after the administration of a medicine that will cause the symptoms to disappear, will actually tie his hands against the finding of a remedy that will be suitable to cure. As surely as the voice of the symptoms is hushed, so surely does the physician put out of his way the opportunity for selecting a homœopathic remedy. When the index to the remedy is spoiled the ability of the physician to benefit his patient is destroyed. If you give quinine, go on with it; if you give an opiate, go on with it; do not go back into Homœopathy. This man who does these things is a homœopathic failure. Some men are incapable of grasping the homœopathic doctrines, and fall into mongrelism, which is a cross between Homœopathy and Allopathy. I would prefer an allopath to one who professes to be a homœopath, but does not know enough Homœopathy to practice it.

Why should you put crude medicines upon the diphtheritic membrane in addition to giving your remedy? If the crude drugs do anything they will spoil the appearance of the throat, and you will not be able to know what your remedy has done. If these adjuvants to the remedy do anything at all they will effect such changes, as will damage the case; if they do not effect changes, why use them? There can be no reason for administering something that does not effect changes. This question came up one time, and created controversy in an association meeting. One doctor recommended the use of Peroxide of Hydrogen in pus cavities; he said it did no harm, it did no damage. The question is, does it do anything at all? If it does, the changes it effects injure the case.

Lay it down, as a rule, that you will use nothing that can effect changes in a case in addition to your remedy. After you prescribe a remedy you want to know when you come back whether that remedy has done anything. For this reason you must rest your case upon that which you believe to be the nearest homœopathic remedy. All changes must be watched, because by observing changes we know what next to do. If something has been given by the patient's friends and changes have occurred in the case from such meddling the doctor is in confusion. If absolutely no changes have occurred after his remedy then he is in intelligence and knows what next to do.

Doctors sometimes give opium to suppress pain, but it is more frequently given to suppress the cry of people that stand around listening to the patient. The friends stand there wringing their hands and saying: "Doctor, cannot you do something?" and the poor doctor loses his head and gives a dose of opium. What does he do that for? In order to quiet the cry of the people. He knows he is damaging his patient, he knows he has put out of his hands the ability to cure that patient homœopathically. What if the patient does suffer? Can that be an excuse for the doctor destroying his power to heal that patient hereafter? The doctor justifies himself by saying, "If I had not done this the people would have criticized me." What business is it of the people? If a doctor has not the grit to withstand the cries of the family, the criticisms of the friends, the threatening of his pocketbook and of his bread and butter, he will not practice Homœopathy very long. An honest man does not fear these things. There is but one thing for him to consider, what is the right thing he must do. The harangue of the crazy old women who stand around wagging their tattling tongues. what has that to do with the life of the patient or the duty of the patient or the duty of the physician? Will they shoulder the responsibility of the patient's death, if he die? I say now that the death of a patient is nothing in comparison with violation of the law on the part of the doctor. In both instances the doctor gets the worst of it. The doctor who violates the law also violates his conscience. and his death is worse than the death of the patient. Generally the physician who has knowledge enough and grit enough to wait will see, before the patient dies, the homœopathic remedy that will control the case. The whole community is sometimes turned into excitement because a doctor will not do this or that. Suppose the whole atmosphere is blue with effects of their wrath, what has that to do with it? The physician who will stick by the patient and let the people howl is one that will be trusted through any and every ordeal. But the doctor that will flinch and tremble at every threatening is one that will violate his conscience, is one that can be bought, can be hired to do anything, and will abandon his color in time of emergency. It is hard work for a homœopathic physician to settle off alone by himself where he has nobody that will stand by him in his tribulations. The attitude of the public must never furnish the physician with indications as to what he shall do. Let him study the patient and the symptoms of the patient. That which is right is protected and supported, and that which is wrong degrades. Let a man lose his self-respect a few times and he becomes a coward and a sneak, and is ready to do almost anything that is vicious and cowardly. The physician who has done rightly by his patient can look the friends squarely in the face when the patient has died. If he has administered morphine to the patient and turned aside all the symptoms upon which he could find tht remedy, it does not seem to me that he can look the friends squarely in the face. Of course, if you act according to principle in this way you suffer for it. You will be called names.

In the 63rd and 64th paragraphs Hahnemann treats of the primary and secondary actions of medicines. There is no necessity for dwelling upon this subject. The primary and secondary actions of a drug are simply the one action of that drug. Some homœopaths have attempted to individualize between the primary and secondary action. It does not matter what the patient is suffering from, from symptoms which appeared in the primary action or from symptoms which appeared in the secondary action, that drug will cure just the same. The symptoms that arise are the symptoms that arise from the remedy, and they often seem to oppose each other. In the earlier stages we have sometimes sleeplessness; in the last stages, sleepiness, and one state is sometimes more prominent than the other. For instance in Opium, some provers had sleeplessness first and sleepiness afterwards, from the smaller doses of Opium. It is known that Opium has both sleeplessness and sleepiness, and if the other symptoms agree it does not matter which one of the two is present. If Opium is indicated by the general state of the patient it will cure either of these conditions, and you need not stop to see if it produces one state in one place and the opposite in another. In some provers Opium produces diarrhœa in the beginning, in others constipation. If I should take today a crude dose of Opium, in six hours I would have a diarrhœa that would last for several days and then be constipated for six weeks. To know that drugs have two actions is simply knowing the nature of drugs in general. You will find another example in alcohol; watch two drunkards and you will see the double action illustrated.

There are constitutional states in patients by virtue of which they are always affected in a certain way, and these states are often left after provings, or are found in those who have been poisoned by a drug. All these patients will have alternating symptoms which will confuse the physician before he knows their constitutional state. It is an important thing to know the constituional state of a patient before prescribing. You will always be able to do better for your patients when you know all of their tendencies. Of course, in acute diseases symptoms sometimes stand out so sharply that an acute remedy can be administered without reference to any constitutional state. Acute cognates can be established in almost any patient. For instance, the Calcarea patient will need an acute cognate of Calcarea when he is sick with acute symptoms. The acute symptoms fit into and are established and formed by the constitutional state of the patient.

LECTURE XVII

THE SCIENCE AND THE ART

Up to this time we have been studying principles that relate to the knowledge of Homœopathy. At this point Hahnemann arrives at three important conclusions as to what we have been studying in application to practice. There are three steps to be surveyed:

1st. "By what means is the physician to arrive at the necessary information relative to a disease, in order to be able to undertake the cure?" Of course that relates to the disease in general, and the patient in particular. In going over the 3rd paragraph, we gathered together the means of studying an epidemic and each man in particular. We shall now proceed to study disease in general and the patient in particular, from now on to the end of this course. All the rest of the study is of such a character. There are a great many questions that arise in this problem that must be studied in detail, the study of the nature of acute miasms and the study of the nature of chronic miasms; the study of such changes as show there are two distinct classes of sickness. Each one is to be studied in its most general way, and each person as a particular entity.

2d. "How is he to discover the morbific powers of medicines; that is to say, of the instruments destined to cure natural disease?" This constitutes a study of the Materia Medica and a knowledge of how it is built, which is by provings, by recorded facts.

3d. "What is the best mode of applying these morbific powers (medicines) in the cure of diseases?" This involves the study of all methods and settling upon that which is best.

To proceed in the study of these in a rational, scientific and careful manner is the object of the future study of this book. It leads, from now on, from the science of Homœopathy to the art of healing. We see that we have now gone over the principal part of that which is merely science, the science of Homœopathy. We have none of the enormous classifications in the study of Homœopathy that are resorted to in traditional medicine; they should not appear in the study of applied Homœopathy. The study of the classification of disease as is done in traditional medicine is useful, because we come in contact with the world. As the Boards of

Health require us to state what particular disease, according to classification, a patient died from, classified in accordance with old school nosology, we have therefore, to go into the study of diagnosis. In Homœopathy, diagnosis cuts very little figure in the treatment; but all the ultimates in the case must be brought forward and described by name. We want the use of adjectives, we want the use of large language, we want descriptive power, in order that the nature of the sickness, which is all that man can know about the disease, may be brought out on paper, and thereby caused to appear at any time thereafter to the mind of the physician. If the physician were simply to make a study of the disease, and after studying it were to give it a name and let that name constitute the record, no future prescription could be made. And the physician, thereafter, in referring to this record, would know nothing about its nature. The name conveys no idea of the nature of the sickness, only its place in a general classification. A knowledge of the nature of individual sickness is necessary for a prescription, and this depends upon the ascertainment of the details.

The very first of this study is to prove and realize that there are two classes of diseases, acute and chronic. The general classification of all diseases is made in this way; the acute are thrown into one group and studied as acute diseases, and so with the chronic.

An acute miasm is one that comes upon the economy, passes through its regular prodromal period, longer or shorter, has its period of progress and period of decline, and in which there is a tendency to recovery. A chronic miasm is one that has its period of prodrome, period of progress and no period of decline; it is continuous, never ending, except with the death of the patient.

The acute diseases need much less study than the chronic. They are all such as are contagious or infectious, such as have a miasmatic character and are capable of running a definite course. When man disorders his stomach and has an attack of vomiting, and from which he has no after trouble, he has suffered merely from an indisposition. Such conditions from external causes are not miasms. Things that go through the mouth into the stomach and thereby produce sickness act either as rousers up of some old trouble or as mechanical causes of disturbance. The pure disease, on the other hand, whether acquired or inherited, are those that flow from the innermost to the outermost while making man sick. These causes that make man sick are influx of simple substance and they run a fixed distinct course. Each one has its own time of pro-drome, its own period of progress, whereby the traditional school of medicine has fixed what it calls pathognomonic symptoms. It is well to know these symptoms, not for the purpose of naming merely, but for the purpose of association.

The study of disease should not be for the purpose of naming; if it is so, the name does harm. When you think of a child suffer-ing from measles, the idea of measles may go out of mind, but the character of the sickness of that particular child must remain in the mind. At first you will not be able to see what is meant by that, especially if you have been in the habit of studying cases for the purpose of diagnosis.

I do not say this to throw a cloud upon diagnosis, but to show that the study of diagnosis is not for the purpose of making a pre-scription. The more you dwell upon diagnostic symptoms, the more you will becloud the ideas entering the mind that lead toward a prescription. You might go into the room and work an hour indivi-dualizing a case, deciding whether it were measles or scarlet fever (there are some confusing cases in the beginning). Well, you might say, it is measles, and must now have Pulsatilla, or scarlet fever and must have Belladonna. You will really see that such a state of affairs is misleading to the mind. If you are in an epidemic, where it is necessary in order to save the neighbourhood, to know, for instance, whether a certain case is of cholera or not, then it becomes necessary to do the two things. The family and the surrounding families are entitled to the safety that a correct knowledge would give and that protection, isolation or quarantine would afford. There are two kinds of study, one with a bearing toward the classi-fication that the disease belongs to, and one with reference to the remedy that the patient needs; but I prefer to settle the patient first as to the remedy he needs, and this has very little to do with the classification, except in a general way. After a remedy has been decided upon that clearly covers the symptoms and the patient receives his dose of medicine, the next point is, what step is neces-sary to take in order to protect the people if this is a contagious disease. Diagnosis is something that a physician cannot afford to be foolish about, he cannot afford to be a blunderer, he cannot afford to go around calling scarlet fever measles, and measles scarlet fever. He must know enough about the general nature of diseases that after the prescription has been made and the patient settled as to that, and the mother wants to know what is the matter with the child, to tell her, for, in that instance, she has a perfect right to know; that is, a case where the family must be protected, where outsiders must be protected; the physician must decide whether it is proper for the child to go to school, or whether it is not proper.

There are some conditions of chronic diseases which closely resemble acute diseases; for instance, these mimicking acute attacks that come on regularly as periodical headaches. One attack, singled out, might have the appearance of an acute miasm, yet the tendency to progress and not to recovery shows that it belongs to the chronic class. Those disorders that come from debauchery and drinking and overeating, from immediate circumstances that are periodical, are things that arise from the latent psoric condition; they are momentary sickness, and if it were not for the fact that man suffers from chronic miasms he would not have these; these attacks would not form a sickness, would not have an appearance of acute sickness. It is due to chronic miasms that man has these little recurring attacks. These do not come with a prodromal period, a progressive period and a period of decline; they may have an attack and decline, but not a prodrome. The acute miasms like the chronic have the prodromal period.

Par. 72 says: "Relative to the first point, it will be necessary for us to enter here into some general considerations. The diseases of man resolve themselves into two classes," etc. Remember that the acute diseases always tend to recovery; the chronic diseases have no tendency whatever to recovery, but a continuous progressive tendency; they are far deeper miasms.

There are three of these chronic miasms that belong to the human family—psora, syphilis and sycosis—and these we will take up and study. The worst cases are those wherein the three chronic miasms, or some parts of the three, have been complicated by drugs. When the effect of drugs has been removed then we may begin to study the pure miasms themselves, but the miasms are complicated at the present day in most men, for whenever we come in contact with chronic sickness we come in contact also with chronic drugging and its effect upon the vital force. I am of the opinion, perhaps I am wrong, that when blood-letting was in vogue, when violent cathartics were thrown in, when emetics and sweating were prescribed, as in the olden times, when all these violent things were resorted to, the human race was not torn to pieces as rapidly as at the present day. The enormous doses of Jalap and Calomel rushed through the intestines and cleaned out the patient, and he felt better afterwards, and probably did not carry to his grave the internal results of that cleaning out. He did not carry the internal results of the emetics and sudorifics, but at the present day small doses of concentrated drugs are administered, which have an insidious effect upon the economy and develop their chronic symptoms very slowly. From the continued taking of old school products, the alkaloids, etc., we have the most dreadful state that has ever occurred in the history of medicine coming on. The aim is to get small doses, to get an insidious effect. The milder preparations, like Sulphonal, require months to develop their chronic tendencies, and are most vicious and troublesome drugs. These slow and subtle preparations are now being manufactured, and though seeming to produce a mild primary effect have secondary effects or after-effects which are very severe. Hahnemann said, in his time, the most troublesome chronic diseases were those that had been complicated with drugs. If that were true then it is ten times so now. The little headache compounds, the catarrh cures, etc., are milder as to the first effects, but more violent as to the last effects. They are prepared to imitate the palatable form of homœopathic remedies.

LECTURE XVIII

CHRONIC DISEASES—PSORA

Psora is the beginning of all physical sickness. Had psora never been established as a miasm upon the human race, the other two chronic diseases would have been impossible, and susceptibility to acute diseases would have been impossible. All the diseases of man are built upon psora; hence it is the foundation of sickness; all other sickness came afterwards.

Psora is the underlying cause, and is the primitive or primary disorder of the human race. It is a disordered state of the internal economy of the human race. This state expresses itself in the forms of the varying chronic diseases, or chronic manifestations. If the human race had remained in a state of perfect order, psora could not have existed. The susceptibility to psora opens out a question altogether too broad to study among the sciences in a medical college. It is altogether too extensive, for it goes to the very primitive wrong of the human race, the very first sickness of the human race, that is the spiritual sickness, from which first state the race progressed into what may be called the true susceptibility to psora, which in turn laid the foundation for other diseases. If we regard psora as synonymous with itch, we fail to understand, and fail to express thereby, anything like the original intention of Hahnemann. The itch is commonly supposed to be a limited thing, something superficial, caused by a little tiny bit of a mite that is supposed to have life, and when the little itch mite is destroyed the cause of itch is said to have been removed. What a folly!

From a small beginning with wonderful progress, psora spreads out into its underlying states and manifests itself in the large portion of the chronic diseases upon the human race. It embraces epilepsy, insanity, the malignant diseases, tumors, ulcers, catarrhs, and a great proportion of the eruptions. It progresses from simple states to the very highest degree of complexity, not always alone and by itself, but often by the villainous aid of drugging during generation after generation; for the physician has endeavored with all his power to drive it from the surface, and has thereby caused it to root itself deeper, to become more dense and invisible, until the human race is almost threatened with extinction. Look at the number of the population upon the face of the earth, and notice how few arrive at the age of maturity. It is appalling to think of the number of infants that die, and these largely from the outgrowths, or outcoming of psora. We see little ones born who have not sufficient vitality to live. The congenital debility, and marasmus, and varying diseases of a chronic character that carry off the little ones have for their underlying cause the chronic miasms. The principal underlying cause is psora, next syphilis and next sycosis.

It required twelve years for Hahnemann to discover and gather together the evidence upon which he came to his conclusions. When a patient came to him who manifested chronic disease in any way he took pains to write down carefully in detail all the symptoms, from beginning to end, with the history of the father and mother, until he had collected a great number of appearances of disease, not knowing yet what the outcome would be; but after this careful writing out of the symptoms of hundreds of patients, little and great, and comparing them and then gathering them together in one grand group, there appeared in the totality of this collection a picture of psora in all of its forms. Up to this time the world had been looking upon each one of these varying forms as distinct in itself, e.g., all the striking features of epilepsy would be gathered together, and epilepsy was then called a disease; but epilepsy is only one of the results of disease, and never appears twice alike. Every person who has epilepsy differs from every other epileptic on earth. But epilepsy, insanity, diabetes, cancer, Bright's disease, and every other case of so-called disease have all had a beginning and one beginning. They are not distinct, but operate in each person in accordance with that individual. Hahnemann says that before he began that collection of symptoms he was struck somewhat with wonder that Nux Vomica and Ignatia and such short acting medicines were able to cure only a single manifestation of disease, a group of symptoms, or they would relieve for a time and then the symptoms would come back, although he had followed up the treatment to the best of his knowledge. At the end of a case, he could discover that there had been a continuous progress in spite of the fact that he had relieved his patient of suffering a good many times.

So it is, while acute acting remedies are used, and you will use them if you do not know the psoric doctrine. The short acting medicines are the ones that contain the counterparts of the acute manifestations of psora, and hence when these acute manifestations appear in groups of symptoms you will naturally select acute remedies, and you will palliate them from time to time, but at the end of years you will look upon every individual case, and will notice that the case has been steadily progressing. You will find that you have not struck at the root of the trouble, that there is an underlying something present and prevailing and that the disease is steadily growing worse.

Hahnemann saw this and it was a mystery to him because he had acquired a perfect mastery over the acute diseases with the acute remedies. Such apsorics had been at this time very well proved, Belladonna, Aconite, Bryonia, Arnica, China, Nux Vomica, etc., etc., and these had been found to be perfectly suitable for the acute manifestations of psora and for the acute miasms. Hahnemann had not yet learned that the acute miasms were utterly and strictly acute miasms; and could not, therefore, compare acute miasms with chronic miasms, or vice versa. He had not seen them yet as miasms.

One will not understand the acute miasms clearly until able to compare them with chronic miasms. They side up one with another, and make it wonderfully manifest. The acute miasms come on either with sufficient violence to cause death to patients, or with less violence, wherein there is a period of progress and a tendency to recover. They cannot be prolonged in the patient, and must subside. The acute miasms are not governed in accordance with fixed time in order to be acute miasms, because they have times of their own. Neither is there a time after the lapse of which the chronic miasm is said to be chronic. According to the old school, diseases have been divided into acute, sub-acute and chronic. If any sickness ran longer than six weeks, it would be placed among the sub-acute; if it ran on indefinitely, it was called chronic. But a chronic miasm is chronic from its beginning, and an acute miasm is acute from its beginning. It is from its nature, from its capabilities, from what it will do to the human race, that we must name the miasm.

So Hahnemann tells us frankly that he was astonished to find at the end of a certain length of time no progress had been made with his remedies in chronic diseases. The symptoms appeared with their own regularity, much stronger than before, which showed they were progressing. Hahnemann enters not only a difficult study, but with all sorts of difficulties, and after studying for twelve years he developed the fact that in all cases observed there was an underlying chronic disease, a chronic miasm, which had a tendency to progress and to end only with the life of the patient. Then he bent himself to the provings of medicines in order to discover from them a likeness to the chronic miasms. Had he never come to this conclusion, he would not have noticed such things.

When he had brought all the symptoms before the mind in one grand collective view, he began to observe and reflect as to what was the first, and what was the second, and later appearances in the line of progress in this deep-seated chronic miasm. Thus it was that he observed amongst those who were dying with phthisis that in their younger days they had a vesicular disease between the fingers and upon the body, which had been suppressed by the ointments in vogue at that time. Then the question naturally arose, what had this suppression to do with that which came afterwards? As to how Hahnemann figured out the answer to that question you can read in his "Chronic Diseases," but he does not tell it all; although he gives many pages of experiences and observations. You will more clearly understand and be better prepared to take up Hahnemann's line of thinking, if you enter into the use of appropriate medicines and apply principle to the progress of disease that is, you will see a demonstration of his teaching in the curative treatment of a very large number of cases of sickness by applying principles : that diseases get well in the reverse order of their coming, that the latest symptoms will be the first to go away, and that the older symptoms will come and go in reverse order in which they appeared; old symptoms, in the form of eruptions, come back, old chills, which have been suppressed, come back, and many other chronic manifestations come back again in a sort of successive order. If we observe these things we must come to the conclusion that when we have driven these oldest and deepest troubles back to their original manifestations, which was perhaps a vesicular eruption, and if we see nothing more simple than this eruption, we must conclude that the suppression of such an eruption was the beginning of trouble.

If you practice accurately, you will observe these things; if you are not a success in practice, you will not observe these things. Many patients are so badly off that this is never observed, and then we have the onward progress; that is, we have the patient declining, instead of the disease declining. If that patient is only better as to symptoms, and his old symptoms do not come back, we know that he is only being palliated, that the disease processes are only being restrained, but that it is not a case of cure. There is one thing that you should know and it is sometimes best to say it to the patient, and that is that they should not take too much courage, because a patient that takes too much courage may take too much discouragement when reverses come. So when a woman walks into your office and says beautiful things by way of gratitude for what you have done for her, because you have mitigated the deep-seated trouble, perhaps chronic sick headache, or epilepsy, but she cannot tell you of an eruption returning or you have observed no backward progress of that disease, no reverse order of the symptoms, it is often well to say to that patient, that not-withstanding the fact that she appears to be much improved the trouble is not over for all that. On the other hand, it is sometimes wise to say: "If an eruption should come out, do not on your life meddle with it," because they will probably use what they say relieved it in the first place, some Sulphur ointment, or some other miserable stuff. The physician should bear in mind to caution the patient against removing any of the symptoms in the case. When the patient comes and reports such wonderful tales of progress, take down your record and look it over. If you have in the record failed to get the earlier history of the case, endeavour then, if possible, to find out something about the previous symptoms, the earlier symptoms, and then it is sometimes well with an intelligent person to say: "Do not be surprised, do not be alarmed, if such and such symptoms return," cautioning the patient to report to the physician and apply nothing. Now, it is from these circumstances that we observe finally, where the patient is so well instructed not to do anything, to take no drugs, to keep the life as pure as possible, to keep the physical forces untrammeled by violence, it is under such circumstances that we shall observe the coming back of symptoms that have long been suppressed. Long after the treatment has ceased, a patient will come back and say: "This old trouble has come back on me; can you do anything for it?" You have now to look over the record, and you see that sure enough this is like what came out in the beginning of this trouble; that psora existed in its simplest form of a vesicular eruption upon the child, and that it was suppressed.

These are the simplest cases of psora, because these can be counted collectively in one person; but the complicated forms of psora are those that are inherited. Amongst the simple forms of psora, after the eruptions disappear, catarrhal troubles come on, with their varying manifestations. You prescribe for all these symptoms, and presently the eruptions of childhood come back, especially in a younger person. If it is in a more complicated state, we do not get the patient back to the original form of psora, because the parent had the simple form of psora, and the child gets a complex form from those which were present when tho patient came to you. You will seldom see the vesicular form or simple form brought back except in those who have had the simple form, but forms approximating the simple will return if the vital energy of the economy is being turned into order.

Since this, then, is the natural form of economy, we see we are gradually travelling back towards the beginning of psora or its earlier forms. If you are treating a vicious form of scaly eruptions, dry hard horney scales, you will, under accurate prescribing, notice these scaly formations disappear, but after the vital force has become strong enough you need not be surprised to see *vesicular* eruptions develop, for the original so-called disease had changed from its vicious squamos form to the milder vesicular form. Different names have been given to the skin diseases, but we see that names are of very little value. The different eruptions change into varying forms but they are all from one cause, and will come back in their successive stages under true homœopathic treatment. This is seen quite often enough to demonstrate what I am talking about, and from this alone we can ascertain that psora begins with the simple isolated vesicular form of eruption. At times you will be treating the more advanced and complicated forms of psora, where there are organic changes; after the patient gets the homœopathic remedy for a while he comes to a standstill, seems to be doing nothing, but in the course of time vicious ugly eruptions come out upon the body. This is a good sign in so far as the disease manifests itself upon the skin, or in catarrhal discharges, the internal organs are safe, but when these outward manifestations are stopped the internal parts suffer.

If this be true, what conclusion must we come to as to the good or injury done to patients when every catarrhal discharge is stopped and every eruption upon the skin is driven away by outward applications? What are we to conclude when we see that the idea of the medical world of today is to stop everything that appears upon the surface? When we know the truth in regard to psora, we see what a wonderful damage it is to the patient to have these outward signs stopped in this way, what a tremendous shock it is to the economy, and how it is that psora is pushed on and made worse, made more complex from year to year, from generation to generation, until it is the fundamental disease of the human economy and the basis of all the trouble in man.

At the present day, as you are now prepared to hear, we can really learn more about psora by watching it in its backward progress than by watching it in its onward progress in any particular case. It is the cause of the chronic manifestations of disease that are not syphilitic or sycotic. We are able to group together in the mind all those vicious constitutional states (not syphilitic or sycotic) that are called organic disease, as the results of psora. Then the five forms of Bright's disease are not diseases, but the result of psora operating upon the economy and attacking the kidney. The common chronic diseases of the liver are not diseases, but the localization of psora in the liver; the lung diseases and heart diseases and brain diseases are not diseases, because they have one single origin, and from this origin we follow their progress and thus study them from their beginnings to their ends, from cause to ultimates. Only in this way will we have a clear knowledge of their internal cause and beginnings.

LECTURE XIX

CHRONIC DISEASES—PSORA (Continued)

In the work on "Chronic Diseases" Hahnemann refers to psora as the oldest, most universal and most pernicious chronic miasmatic disease, yet it has been misappropriated more than any other. "Psora is the oldest miasmatic chronic disease known. The oldest history of the oldest nation does not reach its origin. Psora is just as tedious as syphilis and sycosis, and is, moreover, hydra-headed. Unless it is thoroughly cured, it lasts until the last breath of the longest life. Not even the most robust constitution, by its own unaided efforts, is able to annihilate and extinguish psora."

The three chronic miasms, psora, syphilis and sycosis, are all contagious. In each instance there is something prior to the manifestations which we call disease. We speak of the signs and symptoms of a disease, we speak of the outcroppings of the symptoms when we speak of syphilis, but remember there is a state prior to syphilis or syphilis would not exist. It could not come upon man except for a condition suitable to its development. In like manner psora could not exist except for a condition in mankind suitable for its development.

Psora being the first and the other two coming later, it is proper for us to inquire into that state of the human race that would be suitable for the development of psora. There must have been a state of the human race suitable to the development of psora; it could not have come upon a perfectly healthy race, and it would not exist in a perfectly healthy race. There must have been some sickness prior to this state, which we recognize as the chronic miasm psora; some state of disorder, some state that it would be perfectly rational and proper for man to undertake to solve as to its cause, as to its history, and as to its very nature. Some will say, but if we undertake to do this we will have to accept the word of God as historical, as relating to the beginning, because there is no other going so far back. There is no harm in reasoning from that and I hope you will so accept it, not only as history, but as divine revelation, not that I wish to quote from or refer to it, because I never do so in my teaching. If we look upon syphilis we will see that man's own act leads him to the place where he comes in contact with syphilis; it is the result of action.

Sypilis is that disease which corresponds to the effect of impure coition, of going where syphilis is, of coming in contact with those who have it. It is an action; it is not so with psora. Man does not seek it, he does not go where it is, he does not associate with those necessarily that have it. He may be exposed; but syphilis is the result of his own action, which is an impure fornication or adulteration which he knows better than to seek, and knows enough from his intelligence to avoid. Syphilis, then, is a result of action, although after once ultimated it may be perpetuated by accident. There is always a state and condition of man that precedes his action, and if syphilis corresponds to man's action, and there is a state prior to it, a diseased condition that precedes, that state must correspond to that which precedes action, which is thinking and willing.

Thinking and willing establishes a state in man that identifies the condition he is in. As long as man continued to think that which was true and held that which was good to the neighbor, that which was uprightness and justice, so long man remained upon the earth free from the susceptibility to disease, because that was the state in which he was created. So long as he remained in that state and preserved his integrity he was not susceptible to disease and he gave forth no aura that could cause contagion; but when man began to will the things that were the outcome of his false thinking then he entered a state which was the perfect correspondence of his interior. As are the will and understanding, so will be the external of man. As the life of man or as the will of man, so is the body of man, and as the two make one in this world, there is evolved from him an aura which is vicious in proportion to his departure from virtue and justice into evils. And long before the time of Noah's flood, which was an inundation that destroyed the evil ones that were upon the earth at that time, there was a manifestation, called leprosy, which was but the result of the dreadful profanity that took place in this period. A great many people suffered then from the violent aura of leprosy, whereas the natural disorder of the human race today is a milder form of psora upon a different race of people. If we had the same race upon the earth today we would have leprosy among them, as we now have the milder form of psora. The ancients referred to leprosy as an internal itch.

Hence this state, the state of the human mind and the state of the human body, is a state of susceptibility to disease from willing evils, from thinking that which is false and making life one continuous heredity of false things, and so this form of disease, psora, is but an outward manifestation of that which is prior in man. It was not due to actions of the body, as we find syphilis and sycosis to be, but due to an influx from a state, which progressed and established itself upon the earth, until we can see it as but the outward manifestations of man's very nature.

The human race today walking the face of the earth is but little better than a moral leper. Such is the state of the human mind at the present day. To put it another way, everyone is psoric. We know what leprosy means, and to say that the whole world is in a state of psora is no broader or narrower than to say that leprosy prevails today upon the face of the earth, but it prevails in a milder form, in the form of psora. A new contagion comes with every child. As Psora piles up generation after generation, century after century the susceptibility to it increases. This is true of every miasm and true of all drugs. We find in the drugged world that those who have been mercurized become more susceptible to Mercury and are more easily poisoned by it. Those poisoned with Rhus are so sensitive to it that they cannot go within a whiff of it; those that have been poisoned in their earliest beginning with psora become more sensitive to it, so that in childhood the slightest whiff of it from their school friends will bring on a crop of vesicles between the fingers attended with the acarus.

Of course, some persons will say that the acarus is prior to the eruption, but they don't know that a healthy person will not be affected by the acarus. The miasm is simply evolved out of a state and the acarus is in turn its ultimate. It is the state that is prior, the itching is not prior. The human race becomes increasingly sensitive generation after generation to this internal state, and this internal state is the underlying cause which predisposes man to syphilis. If he had not psora he could not take syphilis; there would be no ground in his economy upon which it would thrive and develop.

The will and the understanding are prior to man's action. This is fundamental. The man does not do until he wills; he wills what he carries out. If man did what he did not will, he would be only an automaton. He wills to go to a house of prostitution, or seeks for a prostitute with whom to copulate, and from her he takes the syphilitic miasm. This action of his will and this disease corresponds to the man. There is a state in which he thinks it only, in which he wills, but in which he has not yet arrived at the state in which he can act. First there was the thinking of falses and willing of evils, thinking such falses as led to depraved living and long for what was not one's own, until finally action prevailed. The miasms which succeeded psora were but the outward representations of actions, which have grown out of thinking and willing.

Psora is the oldest outward expression of the diseases of the human race representing this vital beginning, and next exists that state that corresponds to action. Thinking, willing and acting are the three things that make up the science of the life of the human race. Man thinks, he wills and he acts. Now, that aura which is given out from the human race at any period of its history is that which corresponds to the state of the human race. The children inherit it from their parents and carry it on and continue it. As the internal is so is the external, and the external cannot be except as the result of the internal.

The internal state of man is prior to that which surrounds him; therefore, environment is not cause; it is only, as it were, a sounding board; it only reacts upon and reflects the internal. One who has the prior, which is internal, may have that which can follow upon the external; it flows, as it were from the internal and effects its forms upon the skin, upon the organs, upon the body of man. Such is influx and the inflowing is always in the direction of the least or no resistance; so that it is in the direction of man's affections, man's loves. Things flow in the direction he wants them to flow. Diseases correspond to man's affections, and the diseases that are upon the human race today are but the outward expression of man's interiors, and it is true if the diseases are such they represent the internal forces of man. Man hates his neighbour, he is willing to violate every commandment; such is the state of man today. This state is represented in man's diseases. All diseases upon the earth, acute and chronic, are representations of man's internals. Otherwise he could not be susceptible, or could not develop that which is within him. The image of his own interior self comes out in disease.

This state has continued to progress, and it has accumulated and become complex. The original simple psora has added to it syphilis and sycosis, and these progress and have now effected a state, they have continued to effect a state in mankind, whereby the race is so susceptible to acute affections that many of our citizens have every little thing that comes along, and every little epidemic of influenza brings them down with an acute attack. This could not be but for the complications that a man has caused himself to get into, or has taken upon himself. This was not done in one generation, but has been accumulating upon the face of the earth so long as we have a history of man. Otherwise man would not be sick, for he should be a perfect animal in his animal nature. Look at the perfection of all things put upon the earth; see the plants, how perfect they are; but man by his thinking evils and willing falses has entered upon a state wherein he has lost his freedom, his internal order, and is undergoing changes which the animal kingdom in its period, and the vegetable kingdom in its period, did not take on.

The miasms that are at the present day upon the human race are complicated a thousandfold by allopathic treatment. Every external manifestation of the miasm has in itself a tendency to straighten mankind, but the human race is being violently damaged and diseases are being complicated for the reason that these outward expressions are forced to disappear by the application of some violent or stimulating drug. At the present day nobody will acknowledge that he had the itch in his childhood, until it is seen by some intelligent mother that it is wise to tell the doctor everything. The itch is looked upon as a disgraceful affair; so is everything that has a similar correspondence; because the itch in itself has a correspondence with adultery, only one is adultery as to internal and the other to externals, one succeeds the other. So it is with all miasms.

And now we have the great miasms before us to treat, as physicians, in all their complications. For instance, if a true sycotic gonorrhœa appears to us second hand it appears in its suppressed form, which is a thousand times worse than the original form. All the outward manifestations have been made to disappear. So it is with the external forms of psora, the vesicular and squamous eruptions, and all the outgrowths and outcroppings of psora. Every conceivable thing has been resorted to to destroy its manifestations, and the disease has grown and grown until nobody can tell what its outcome will be. How long can this thing go on before the human race will be swept from the earth with the results of the suppression of psora? From the suppression of psora we have cancerous affections, organic diseases of the heart and lungs, phthisis, and general destruction of the body. How long can it go on? If Homœopathy does not spread, if it does not establish its doctrines upon the earth so that sick folks can be headed under its principles, this threatening state and condition will increase. Allopathic physicians are multiplying rapidly, and they are all doing the same thing, even more so now than at the time of Hahnemann. It does seem as if Homœopathy had become a necessity, but the kind of Homœopathy that is preached in the majority of our schools will not check the progress of psora. The majority of the college teachers sneer at the doctrine of psora; they sneer at the miasms and continue in their efforts to establish Homœopathy upon an allopathic basis. Homœopathy as taught in the colleges at the present day is simply an attempt to establish Homœopathy upon an allopathic basis, using allopathic names, calling chronic affections by different names, and treating diseases of organs by name. No study is made of psora, but allopathic books are their textbooks. Syphilis is not treated from cause to effect, but simply in the way of driving it back or holding it in abeyance, without any effort to permanently cure it. The patient is filled with Mercury, the Iodides and other strong drugs, drugs that are well known to subdue it temporarily by an allopathic effect.

Psora has progressed until it has become the most contagious of diseases, because the more complicated it becomes the more susceptible are our children to its beginnings, and its contagion adds to the old disease; and while it goes on the children become increasingly sensitive to the other miasms. The human race at the present day is intensely susceptible to psora, to syphilis and sycosis. "Psora," says Hahnemann, "became, therefore, the common mother of man's chronic diseases. It can be said that at least seven-eighths of the chronic maladies existing at the present day are due to psora."

True, if psora could be brought back in a series to its simple state the external of the body would become wonderfully bad to look upon, but the internal would be in a much better state. The vesicular eruptions that come are sometimes dreadful to look upon, horrible in proportion to the vanity of the patient, but these must be allowed to evolve themselves and then wonderful good comes to the economy. Hereditary states roll out in these manifestations, internal evils flow into external manifestations and Homœopathy continues to drive them outward and outward, thereby leaving the economy in a state of comparative freedom. Very commonly itch will not yield to the homœopathic treatment immediately, because the action of the remedy is routing the heredity within, causing it to flow out more exteriorily into manifestations without. One who does not know this, of course, loses heart when his remedies do not at once wipe out the eruption. A sickly child may come out with eruptions, and if the child is treated properly the sickness will flow out into the eruption and that child will be cured from within out; and finally after much tribulation the outward trouble will pass away, carrying with it the internal trouble. So that when it is said that the appropriate remedy did not immediately wipe off the skin and make it smooth, and, therefore Zinc ointment or Sulphur ointment was resorted to, we see that it is a violation of law, and a wonderful damage to the patient.

Then Hahnemann gives a long list of cases with authorities, quotations and references which you should certainly look over. He also gives the symptoms that he collected while observing and investigating. It was the wonderful similarity between those symptoms when grouped together, representing an image of psora, and those symptoms representing, an image of Sulphur, which led Hahnemann to the use of Sulphur in psoric conditons. In psora we have the images of many remedies; all of the deep acting remedies have more or less something of the nature of psora.

LECTURE XX

CHRONIC DISEASES—SYPHILIS

There are some generals that relate to this disease under homœo-pathic treatment. It can be found from books what to expect in this disease; for instance, the different syphilitic eruptions in all their varied manifestations as to time and color. In regard to the prodromal period, it is well to remember that it is usually from twelve to fifteen days, but it is sometimes as late as 50 or 60 days. Some acute miasm or a bad cold, or a drug disturbing the economy, may prevent the external manifestations and prolong the prodromal period, but it is usually from 12-15 days, if in no way disturbed or interrupted. Now the prodromal period increases with the conta-gion of the various stages. This is an observation that you will be able to verify in homœopathic practice, but one that the books will not give. The books speak of the primary contagion as the only contagion in connection with the syphilitic miasm, but let me tell you something. Suppose we assume that the syphilitic miasm is a disease that would run for a definite time, and suppose that an individual has gone through with the primary manifestation and is told by his physician that he can safely marry; if he marry, his wife becomes an invalid; but she does not go through the primary manifestations, the initial lesion and the roseola, but she has the syphiloderma and the symptoms which belong to the later stage of the disease. This disease is transferred from husband to wife, and it is taken up in the stage in which it then exists and from thence goes on in a progressive way. The woman catches it from the man in the stage in which he has it at the time of their marriage; she takes that which he has; if he has it in the advanced stage she takes it in that stage; she takes from him the stage he has to offer.

This is equally true of psora and sycosis. Such things never occur in the acute miasm, but the three chronic miasms have contagion in the form in which they exist at the time. The state is trans-ferred, so that one in the advanced stages of psora will transfer to his good wife the psora which he has, and she takes it up and pro-gress with it and adds it to her own, and it progresses in accord-ance with her peculiarities.

But the law of protection by dissimilars often comes in here and saves the wife's system from receiving a new infection of either syphilis, psora or sycosis. The disorders already present in her economy may be so wholly dissimilar that they protect her from contagion. Thus it is that a woman may have coition with a man that has sycosis in the form of gleet, and yet not have it indicated upon her; thus she may have protection against form of chancre. She may remain in contact with him as wife, and even have a child by him, and that child be black with syphilis, while she has no symptoms of syphilis. The reason of that is that the child is from the seed of the father and the mother only furnishes the groundwork.

There are plenty of physiological facts that demonstrate these things. I have seen several cases where the child was born black with syphilis, and have looked for the mother to come down with syphilitic symptoms, but no trace of it could be observed. When infection takes place in the primary stage there is no way of disguising it, but if it occurs in the secondary or tertiary stage there is really no way of detecting it immediately, because it goes on insidiously. If the husband has the primary sore the primary sore will manifest itself in the wife, but if he gives the disease to his wife in the tertiary stage, with every manifestation suppressed or passed by, then you will not be able to know whether she has taken the disease or not. We have already seen in studying the *Organon* that when the diseases are dissimilar to each other one repels the other; so that if the woman has something in her economy in the form of a chronic disease, perhaps a phthisical condition, she will be protected. The organic results are such that the body is overwhelmed with the disease that it already has, and hence she is protected. Dissimilars repel each other, and similars attract and cure each other. Yet if the dissimilar psoric manifestation is of a milder type, and can be substituted by the contagion, then the syphilitic condition comes in. To know the action of diseases upon each other is essential, because we see the principle of cure in how one disease affects another.

We learn much concerning the syphilitic miasm under the action of homœopathic remedies. At the end of the prodromal period we may expect the chancre; at the end of about six weeks, more or less, we may expect the external manifestations, the roseola and other eruptions; soon succeeding these, at the time of their disappearance, or in connection with them, we have the mucous patches in the throat, ulcers in the throat, and finally the falling of the hair. These rapidly succeed each other, often being associated. These are the commonest outward manifestations of the earlier period of secondary syphilis; it is important to remember this. In weakly subjects these come on very feeble; in robust, vigorous constitutions these manifestations come on vigorously. Now it matters not whether the feeble constitution fails to throw these out, or whether because of drugs the constitution has been made feeble and thereby the manifestations are withdrawn when they have been thrown out. The state is the same, whether they are suppressed or withheld because of feeble constitution, *i.e.*, the disease is operating upon the internal, having a tendency to affect the organs that are of the interior man, the brain, the liver, the kidneys, the spleen, the heart and lungs, the tissue and the bones. As syphilis commences to occupy the interior tissues of man the periosteum, the bone and the brain are tissues that are sought out as the principal sites. If you will contrast that with psora you will see that the latter more commonly attacks the blood vessels and the liver and causes deposits beneath the skin, forming suppuration and boils. The syphilitic boil is not a true boil, it is a multiple tubercular mass most vicious in character.

If we observe the syphilitic miasm in its backward progress we will trace it back in its stages, supposing they had been suppressed. In the earlier state the homœopathic treatment strikes at the root of the evil, and will take hold of that which would become latent, and will so turn things into order that the chance that is painful will become painless, will continue on as a mild and harmless sore. The bubo will be hastened to suppuration when it would not otherwise suppurate. The mucous patches will be checked, the sore throat will be greatly relieved, so that the patient is made more comfortable in all of his manifestations. In this earlier state we do not see the backward progress in the form of ulcers, etc., but we see that the tendency of the homœopathic remedy is, as it were, to quiet manifestations or subdue them, until the remedy has taken a deep and permanent hold of the economy, then they gradually subside.

So much for the action of homœopathic remedies upon earlier manifestations. But now if we proceed to examine the very latest manifestations we will see an opposite state. If you take hold of a case that is very late, say an old case that has been five or ten years going the rounds, getting all sorts of vicious treatment, and the patient has those awful biparietal head pains, he is becoming weaker in mind, he is getting the tertiary manifestations in general, tendency to gummatous formations and deep-seated ulcerations, and is threatening to break down in health. You will find constitutional remedies can only restore him and cure him by bringing out external manifestations upon his body somewhere. Not that the primary sore will come back right away; he may never have it at all; but he will begin to have ulcerated sore throat, which may progress and eat all the soft tissues in view, including the soft palate. If this ulceration appears the bones that have been so painful and threatened to become necrosed will cease to be affected; the periostitis will subside. Iritis is likely to be a troublesome symptom and may come with the secondary symptoms, or long years afterwards with tertiary symptoms. The proper remedy will immediately relieve this last appearing symptom, but the patient will say: "Doctor, I wish you would look in my throat; I have not had this trouble for a long time." You see upon examining his throat a mucous membrane that has been sacrificed by the application of Nitric acid and other caustics, indurated, hard, gristly-like tissues that are infiltrated with gummatous deposits. Now, he is in a pickle, for just as sure as he lives that man will have to undergo much trouble if you save him from insanity. If you save him at all, so that he is worth living, these suppressed manifestations must come back, and they will come back under appropriate treatment.

LECTURE XXI

CHRONIC DISEASES—SYCOSIS

It is not generally known that there are two kinds of gonorrhœa, one that is essentially chronic, having no disposition to recovery, but continuing on indefinitely and involving the whole constitution in varying forms of symptoms, and one that is acute, having a tendency to recover after a few weeks or months. They are both contagious. There are also simple inflammations of the urethra attended with discharges which are not contagious, and thus we have simple inflammations of the urethra and specific inflammations of the urethra, and of the specific we have the two kinds I have mentioned, the chronic and acute. The books will treat of them as one disease, treat them in a class, and in a treatise on gonorrhœa we will have a description only of that which relates to the beginning, viz.; the discharge. The majority of the cases of gonorrhœa are acute, *i.e.*, there is a period of prodrome, a period of progress and a period of decline, being thus in accordance with the acute miasms. The acute may really and truly be called a gonorrhœa, because about all there is of it is this discharge. If the suppressive treatment be resorted to in the acute, the system is sufficiently vigorous in most cases to throw off the after effects. The suppression cannot bring on the constitutional symptoms called sycosis. It cannot be followed by fig warts, nor constitutional states, such as anæmia. But while constitutional symptoms cannot follow the suppression of the acute miasm, they will follow suppression of the chronic miasm, and become very serious. Most of the cases of true sycosis that are brought before the physician at the present time are those that have been suppressed, and they are a dozen times more grievous than when in the primary stage.

In both the acute and chronic, the prodromal period is about the same, from eight to twelve days, and there is no essential difference between the discharge of the acute and chronic. It is a mucopurulent discharge, and may have all the appearances that any acute discharge of the urethra might take on. Any simple remedy conforms to the nature of the discharge itself will soon turn the acute miasm into a state of health, but it requires anti-sycotic remedies (remedies that conform to the nature of sycosis) to turn the constitutional sycotic gonorrhœa into health. In the very earliest stage of the discharge it is not necessary to make a distinction; but after the disease progresses for weeks, it becomes necessary to make a distinction, and to follow the remedy that conformed to the more acute symptoms with the remedy that would be suitable in a sycotic constitution fully developed. Remedies are picked out for sycosis in the same way that the remedies are picked out in any miasmatic disease, viz., by making an anamnesis.

An anamnesis of all the sycotic cases which we have had enables us to look at the constitutional state of sycosis just in the same way as Hahnemann, by an anamnesis of psora, ascertained its nature and worked out the remedies that are similar in nature and action to psora. All medicines that are capable of producing the image of sycosis may be called anti-sycotics, but we can put it in this way also and say all those remedies are anti-sycotic which when given to a sycotic case in its advanced state are able to turn the disease backward, to reproduce the earlier forms and bring back the discharge. That is the practical way of demonstrating that a medicine is an anti-sycotic. When it conforms to the image of the miasm, it will turn the disease on its backward course. Those remedies that conform only to a particular part of the case are not deep enough nor similar enough to establish a return to earlier symptoms, and hence they are not truly anti-sycotic.

It is hardly necessary to go over a description of the acute form of gonorrhœa, but let us turn our attention solely to sycosis, recognizing it as a chronic miasm, or a disease whose first stage is a discharge from the urethra. These cases I have said are rare in proportion to the large number of cases of acute gonorrhœa, but the disease seems to be on the increase. Every busy physician will see a good many cases in women and children. Cases of gonorrhœa that have been suppressed by injections in the hands of the old school are considered ended, and soon after the discharge has stopped the sycotic patient may be told by his physician that he is a fit subject to marry as he has been cured. But it is not true, and he should delay marriage. It is not right for him to marry until the discharge has been brought back again, and he has been cured, not by injections, because they only suppress, but by the indicated anti-sycotic. Only then may he marry a healthy wife, and she will continue healthy and bring forth healthy children.

You will never know until you get in practice how common it is for a wife to break down, in a year or eighteen months after marriage, with uterine trouble, with ovarian disease, with abdominal troubles, with all sorts of complaints peculiar to the woman; and you will then be surprised on going into the history of her husband (if you are permitted to do so) to discover that in his earlier life he had two or three attacks of gonorrhœa that were treated with Nitrate of Silver or by one of these prescriptions that are carried around in the vest pockets of vicious young men, by injections that are known to stop these discharges. You will not then be surprised if you learn that the man himself has never had a really genuine state of health since that gonorrhœal discharge disappeared. You will look upon what followed that suppression in the man. You will observe what followed the contagion in the woman and to observe these closely constitutes an interesting study.

Sometimes it is so very severe in form, and the trouble comes so soon after the suppression, that there can be no doubt even in the mind of the man himself, that the trouble he is now suffering from relates to the suppression of that discharge. Sometimes they are latent and develop very gradually, and the blood becomes affected, the gradually increasing anæmia comes, the patient being pallid and waxy. What was said in relation to syphilis about contagion in the stage in which the individual has the disease is true in this disease, as also in psora. Here is a common instance. A sycotic patient has been "cured" as far as the discharge is concerned, and now marries for he is told that no harm can come hereafter but shortly afterwards his wife comes down with illness, whereas she had always been a healthy woman before. In the old school there is no recognition of a gonorrhœal condition; nor could the homœopathic physician be sure of this, except for his careful prescribing.

You take a man who has gone from ten to fifteen years with this sycotic trouble. He is waxy, subject to various kinds of fig warts, his lips are pale and his ears almost transparent; he is going into a decline; he has various kinds of manifestations, and these manifestations appear in numerous particulars that we call symptoms. The physician sits down and makes a careful study of the case, and if his perception of it is similar to some long acting, deep acting medicine, and he administers this medicine to the patient, the patient begins to improve. The treatment is kept up, and in the course of weeks or months the patient comes into the office and says: "Doctor, if I had exposed myself I should think I had an attack of gonorrhœa." Now, knowing the diseases get well in the reverse order of coming, you certainly cannot be surprised to hear this story.

On the other hand, however, the trouble may have manifested itself in other mucous membranes of the body, and thus saved the man from his waxiness; he is not so pallid when the condition becomes busy in another region. These catarrhal manifestations may be catarrhal conditions of the eyes, but are commonly catarrhs of the nose. It is not an uncommon thing for a nasal catarrh to be sycotic and to have existed only since the gonorrhœa was suppressed. The catarrh is located in the nose and posterior nares with thick, copious discharge, and in spite of local treatment it has been impossible to suppress it. When the constitution is vigorous enough it will keep up the discharge in spite of the different specific reme-dies that have been administered, but in constitutions that are feeble diseases are easily driven to the centre, leaving the outer-most parts of man. So it is often the case that a man with a thick, yellowish-green discharge from the nose, after a dose of Calcarea, which is an anti-sycotic, one of the deepest in character, has his old discharge brought back, and he says: "Doctor, I am not able to account for this, for I have been nowhere but with my wife." It is time to sit down and tell that man that in his earlier life he had a gonorrhœa, and that its nature was sycotic; for if it had not been of a specific character, it could not have transferred itself to the man's economy, affecting in that way his nose; that it has disappeared from its new site under the action of a truly homœo-pathic prescription, and the original discharge has been brought back, the trouble that he had in the first place. This must be explained to him, and you can now tell him that he is in a position to regain his health, to become well, to get rid of his catarrh; but that if he meddles with that discharge from the penis he will never recover. Just this kind of a case has been seen so often that there it is no longer a doubt about it.

It is in the nature of gonorrhœa to go to the surface in the earlier stage, and so when the catarrh comes on in vigorous constitutions soon after the suppression of the discharge from the urethra it may locate itself in the nose, but if the catarrh does not come on soon the constitution is too weak for the catarrh to represent the disease, and it will be represented on deeper tissues. Bright's disease may come, breaking down of the lungs, breaking down of the liver, rheumatic affection of the worst form, finally killing the patient. It is only in the earlier stages that it becomes catarrhal. The man thinks he is cured and he has escaped the outward manifestations because his constitution is not very vigorous, but the disease goes on into an advanced state until it attacks the blood and he becomes anæmic.

Now, if in this condition he marry, his wife does not get the catarrhal state, because the contagion is contracted in the bladder trouble, but she gets the anæmic state. You may call it a secondary state if you like, but it is really the more interior form of the disease. From this anæmic state it spreads into all functions of the body. The woman does not get the catarrhal state, because the contagion is contracted in the woman at the stage which the husband has reached. If he has passed the catarrhal stage, what she gets is beyond the catarrhal state. She gets fibrinous condition, inflammation of the uterus and the soft tissues, or low grade changes in the kidneys. She may go on and have any of the peculiar constitutional diseases that the woman of today is subject to. It is rather strange that it affects the soft tissues and not the bones. Syphilis affects the soft tissues and the bones. Psora affects the whole economy, nothing escapes; it causes a general breakdown.

Sometimes in the man it does not take the catarrhal form, but produces inflammation of the testes, or it may affect the rectum. Again, if you go to the bedside of a man who has used strong injections for the purpose of suppressing a gonorrhœal discharge, and you find him in bed writhing and turning, tossing and twisting with the pains, and the only relief for him is to keep in continual motion; the pains are tremendous, they are rending and tearing from head to foot; if he can get up he will walk the floor night and day. There is seldom much swelling with this rheumatism; it seems to be along the sheath of the nerves and is relieved by motion. The superficial physician will say, here is a patient relieved by motion, here is a case for Rhus. You give Rhus, and then find it does not do a single thing for the man; but remember, when you have studied sycosis in its innermost nature, Rhus is not an anti-sycotic remedy and will not help this patient in his restlessness; it will not help his awful distress and anxiety. This state will go on, and when it has attacked him so violently his tendons will begin to contract, they will shorten, the muscles of the calves will become sore, the muscles of the thighs will become so sore that they cannot be touched or handled; sometimes there is infiltration of the muscles and hardness, and this soreness extends to the bottom of the feet so that it is impossible for the patient to walk. He is compelled to sit or lie or crawl around on his hands and knees, so violent are some cases. These cases will go on for years. I have known external applications of the allopathic physician to be applied to these sore feet and limbs for weeks and months and even years, and yet they give no relief; but a correct prescription made by a homœopath, carefully taking in account and covering the whole nature of sycosis, will take the soreness out of the feet and bring back the gonorrhœal discharge. The return of the old symptoms means recovery. When the discharge comes back the relief of these horrible symptoms comes, and do not consider any patient cured until the discharge is brought back.

With reference to the woman, in whom you know that the contagion has taken place in the stage in which it existed in the husband, supposing she has inflammation of a fibrinous character and goes into the very worst forms of anæmia, with all the sallowness and waxiness and patchy condition of the skin and the withering and the organic troubles, if a homœopathic prescription be made that is truly anti-sycotic you need not expect that a gonorrhœal discharge will appear in her case; it is not necessary, she can get well without it. If she had no discharge she can get well without its return. The reverse order of the symptoms in her case means only the reverse order of those she has had. She may not have had the primary, but all that that patient has had she must go back through, stage by stage and symptom by symptom. The woman is the most grievous sufferer; she is an innocent person, and when there are anæmic conditions and a going down steadily in the wife that has come on a few years after marriage you should always be suspicious of this disease, at least do not allow it to pass unless you have made a suitable investigation of the matter. Send for the husband, talk to him quietly, tell him you want to know whether he has gone through any of the specific diseases in his younger days that it shall be considered in confidence. When you are the family physician that must be done.

With fear and trembling he will likely tell you the whole story; he has gone into his marriage with a degree of innocence, because he was advised by his physician that what he has had will not affect his wife. When you have discovered this state in the family, watch their children; they will be few, for sycosis very commonly makes a woman sterile, or if she has a few children you will find in them a strong tendency to marasmus in the first year, or in the first or second summer a strong tendency to consumption, or you will find a withering, old appearance of the face. Any one of these three miasms may predispose this child to these things, but when the child is waxy and anæmic, is accustomed to have lienteric stools, has no digestion, when every hot spell brings on complaints that look like cholera-infantum, and it does not grow, does not thrive, you have a right to suspect it is a sycotic case, for sycosis is the most frequent cause.

This disease, you see, does not manifest itself by many eruptions, except those of a warty character; it does not manifest itself by eruptions like syphilis and psora, but operates by bringing about a rheumatic state and an anæmic condition of the blood. It takes hold of the blood first and conforms to the subjects who are advanced in deep-seated troubles, subject to epithelioma. They are especially subject to Bright's disease and to acute phthisis. If they have pneumonia, it is likely to end in a breakdown of some sort in the lungs. If they have any acute disease of a prolonged character, like typhoid, the recovery is always slow.

Manifestly it is a good thing to know the history of a patient, all the peculiarities of the life of a patient. It is important to know whether that patient is syphilitic or sycotic. You know that everybody is psoric, but those that have lived a proper life have escaped the two contagious diseases which man acquires in the first place by his own seeking. When a patient has gone to the end of typhoid or some lingering disease, you know that he is psoric; but if you also know that he is syphilitic, or that he is sycotic, you can conduct his convalescence into a speedy recovery, and if he denies these things you may be puzzled. The sycotic patient may go into a state of do-nothing and decline at the end of a typhoid fever; convalescence will not be established, he will lie with an aversion to food; he does not react, he does not repair, there is no tissue-making, no assimilation; there is no vitality, he lies in a sort of semi-quiescent state; there is no convalescing in the matter. If you know he is a sycotic patient, he must have an anti-sycotic remedy, and then he will begin to rally. If a syphilitic patient, he must have an anti-syphilitic remedy. If neither of these miasms are present, a remedy looking towards his psoric state will cause him to rally. The nature of these cases must be kept in view, you must remember that these chronic miasms are present in the economy and after an acute illness very often have to be fought. If this is not known, many patients will gradually sink and die for apparent want of vitality to convalesce.

Of course, the anti-sycotic treatment for the infant will bring back, as you will readily see, only that stage which the infant began with. It will not bring out a discharge in the infant. The infant has only the interior nature of the disease, and has not the primary and outermost forms of it. You will also remember another thing, that these infants when they grow up are increasingly sensitive to sycosis; that they are already prepared for a sycotic gonorrhœa whenever the first exposure comes. The susceptibility is laid by his inheritance, just as the susceptibility to psora is laid by our parents and the susceptibility to syphilis is laid by our parents. Man can only have one attack in his natural life-time of one of the three chronic miasms; a man cannot take syphilis twice, he cannot take sycosis twice, he cannot take psora twice. This is not known; a man when asked how many times he has had gonorrhœa will say: "About half a dozen times;" but only one of these was sycotic. The sycotic constitution cannot be taken a second time. One attack gives immunity to that person forever after. The offspring becomes increasingly susceptible to all the miasms the more they become developed in the human race. The more they become complicated with each other the more the human race becomes susceptible to acute and epidemic diseases. Now, you have a general survey of the chronic miasms.

LECTURE XXII

DISEASE AND DRUG STUDY IN GENERAL

Part of your study should be to bring before the mind, as fully as possible, the diseases that the human race is subject to. This cannot be done to any great extent from Old School books, as they do not treat of psora, syphilis and sycosis in such a way as to bring the image of the disease before the mind, and only in a limited way the acute miasms are so brought before the mind. The diagnostic or pathognomonic symptoms are brought out for the purpose of distinguishing one disease from the other, but not with the idea of bringing the image of the disease before the mind that it may look like some remedy recorded in the Materia Medica, because that is not the allopathic physician's way of prescribing. It is important to go over the great bulk of the psoric symptoms that Hahnemann has given to obtain as perfect an image as possible of the disease psora. If we take the *Chronic Diseases* and go over them, writing out opposite every symptom that Hahnemann has mentioned as psoric all the remedies that have been found from provings to correspond to these disease symptoms, we shall have before the mind a list of the anti-psoric remedies. It is a good exercise and a good way of preparing for the study of Materia Medica.

Try to master this: Diseases must not be looked upon from a few symptoms that the patient may possess but from all the symptoms that the whole human race brings out. It is just as improper to look upon psora from a few symptoms as it is to look upon a remedy from a few symptoms. Just as you see the image of a remedy from all the symptoms, including the peculiar symptoms, so psora must be considered from its characteristics, the features that constitute psora. Remedies are adjusted as to appearance; the appearances of the remedy expressed in symptoms must be adjusted to the appearances of the disease expressed in symptoms. When you have finished psora, take up sycosis, and spend much time in gathering together all the symptoms that sycotic patients have felt, all their suffering and all the ultimates. Group them as one, and look upon them as one miasm. Then go to the Materia Medica again and make an anamnesis. Take each symptom and place opposite it all the remedies that have produced that symptom. You can readily see that the remedies that run through most strongly will be anti-sycotic remedies, *i.e.*, the remedies that have the essentials of the disease or the nature of sycosis in them.

In the same way make an anamnesis of syphilis. By these means you will bring before your mind the three chronic diseases of the human race, and when this is accomplished in a general way you will be prepared to enter upon their treatment. But remember that the symptoms, when it comes to prescribing for a chronic patient, constitute the whole basis of the prescription; we have not other. We may theorize as much as we have a mind to, but when it comes to the actual application the symptoms must guide to the remedy. There are, however, a good many different ways of looking at the symptoms. It is a very easy thing to become confused over the symptoms and fall into error by taking symptoms that are unimportant. Your study in the Materia Medica will illustrate how you must study disease, as the plan of studying the Materia Medica for the purpose of bringing the image of a remedy before the mind is the plan we must adopt in studying a disease. The physician who can only hold in his memory the symptoms of a disease or a remedy will never succeed as a homœopath. He has not taught himself to think, he has only a mass of particulars, and nothing to tie to. There is no order. It is like a mob.

Here I want to read you a note of Hahnemann's. "Should it, however, be thought sometimes necessary to have names for diseases, in order to render ourselves intelligible in a few words to the ordinary classes when speaking of a patient, let none be made use of but such as are collective. We ought to say, for instance, that a patient has a species of chorea, a species of dropsy, a species of nervous fever, a species of ague," etc. It will lead the mind into heresy if one gets into the custom of speaking from appearances and naming diseases according to the old way. The homœopathic physician must avoid thinking that way. One who has been in the habit of thinking that way must make a great effort to keep the mind from running in that groove. Of course, it would be folly to talk to an old school physician or to a patient in any other words and we can talk to them so, for the sake of conversing but we must know when we speak in such a way that it is only an appearance.

This now brings us to paragraph 83, which takes up the study and examination of the patient and the qualifications necessary for comprehending the image of a disease. You have probably by this time come to the conclusion that an old school prescriber, and perhaps the majority of such as call themselves homœopaths at the present time, are perfectly incompetent to examine a patient, and therefore incompetent to examine Homœopathy, to test it, so as to say whether there is anything in it or not. They have every element of failure and no element of success. It is impossible to test Homœopathy without learning how to get the disease image so before the eye that the homœopathic remedy can be selected. What a natural thing it would be for an allopathic physician to say: "I am going to test Homœopathy. This patient has a case of vomiting, and I will give Ipecacuanha because it produces vomiting." So he gives Ipecac, and the patient keeps on vomiting. He has tested Homœopathy and it is no good! That is the way tests are usually made. I have had physicians tell me that they have tested Homœopathy and it failed; but I know that it was not Homœopathy that failed but the physician who failed. Whenever failure comes it is a failure of the physician and not of the law. This is about the kind of a test that is made today in this enlightened day and age of the world. They have neither the knowledge nor the state of mind to make a test. They do not know what to observe, or how to select a remedy. If we should look up all the remedies that have vomiting we would find a pretty good list, but to make use of that list the mind must be prepared to see which one in it is similar to this individual patient.

"The examination of a particular case of disease, with the intent of presenting it in its formal state and individuality, only demands on the part of the physician an unprejudiced mind, sound understanding, attention and fidelity in observing and tracing the image of the disease, I will content myself in the present instance with merely explaining the general principles of the course that is to be pursued, leaving it to the physician to select those which are applicable to each particular case."

The first statement is that the physician must be of unprejudiced mind. Where are you going to find such a person? If that is essential, there is almost nobody that can examine a case for the purpose of finding a remedy for that case. An unprejudiced mind! At the present day there is almost no such thing as an unprejudiced mind. Go out among the doctors who profess to practice Homœopathy and you will find they are full of prejudice. They will at once commence to tell you what they believe; one believes one thing and another another thing; they all have varying kinds of belief. This does not come from a question of fact, but it comes from what each man has laid down as fact. What each man wants to be so, in his view, is so. That establishes in his mind a state of prejudice, and as no two agree there are many different opinions, the majority of which must be false. Go into anything that you have a mind to and you will find man full of prejudice. This state of prejudice exists in the examination of a patient. The physician goes to the patient prejudiced as to his own theories. He has own ideas as to what constitutes the correct method of examination, and so he does not examine the patient for the purpose of bringing out the truth, the whole truth and nothing but the truth. His prejudices lead him to snap the patient up as soon as he begins to tell his story. He will thump him all over, from head to foot, and then tell him what is the matter with him. A prescription that has no earthly relation to the constitutional state of the patient follows, but no examination has really been made.

It might readily and truthfully be said that the true man has no prejudices. It is certain that the true man is one freest from prejudices, one who can listen, who can examine evidence and who can meditate. What would we think of a judge who would go into a case with strong prejudice? The law provides that a judge cannot sit in judgment over his brother or over his wife, or over his other relatives. In a homœopathic physician an unprejudiced mind can only be attained by learning all the truth and all the doctrines of Homœopathy. If a physician goes in with prejudice for a certain potency or a certain disease, or a prejudice against certain principles, he is not in a rational state, he is not in freedom with the patient and he goes into the examination in ignorance, and if he cannot free himself from prejudice he cannot prescribe. If a man has arrived at a degree of sound understanding concerning the doctrines of Homœopathy, concerning the doctrines of potentization, concerning the doctrines that relate to chronic and acute diseases, concerning the Materia Medica, he goes into it with full freedom, with an intention to examine the case in all its length and breadth, and to listen patiently. He listens to the friends of the patient and he observes without prejudice, with wisdom and with judgment. He must go into the case without forming any judgment whatever until all the witnesses have told their tale and all the evidence is before him. Then he commences to study the whole case. That is doing it without prejudice and for this a sound understanding is necessary, with a clear knowledge of all things relating to the subject and to all of his duties.

If an allopathic physician was to come in and listen to the long examination of a case by a homœopath he would want to know what it was all about. He does not see anything in it, because he has not a knowledge of true materia medica. The homœopath's purpose is to transfer a man's sickness to paper and so find the image of the sickness in the Materia Medica. The allopathic physician could not do that; he could not put the image of the sickness on canvas so that he could fit the picture to the Materia Medica, for he would not know one of our medicines with which to compare it. The unprejudiced mind then comes from sound understanding, and a sound understanding comes from education. The education we are now talking about is an education in Homœopathy, becoming acquainted with all the doctrines step by step. After being taught how to give attention and what to give attention to fidelity is necessary. This faithfulness would never be shown by one who had not removed all his prejudices by opening his mind to the principles and doctrines. Here we work together; we all work after the same fashion. Take everyone of the students that goes through here for a year, and you will find that he has the ways of the school and carries the stamp of the school. Just as the stamp of Harvard or the stamp of Yale is upon every student that comes from either of these institutions so the stamp of the Post Graduate School is upon every student that goes through its curriculum with faithfulness and earnestness.

What we are now about to consider is the plan for the faithful and careful examination of a case. It is our purpose to cure the case, and it is necessary for this purpose to bring the patient's symptoms in the very best possible way before the mind. This is a long and tedious study, and there are many difficulties in the way. Disease must be brought out in symptoms, with the end of its becoming a likeness of some remedy of the Materia Medica. All the diseases known to man have their likeness in the Materia Medica, and the physician must become so conversant with this art that he may perceive this likeness. You will find at first it is not an easy matter and that, to become expert, requires the continual application of patience. All the senses must be on the alert in order to perceive that which is similar, and most similar. Now we come to the directions to the physician for discovering and tracing out the image of the disease.

LECTURE XXIII

THE EXAMINATION OF THE PATIENT

§ 84. The patient details his sufferings; the persons who are about him relate what he has complained of, how he has behaved himself, and all that they have remarked in him. The physician sees, hears and observes with his other senses whatever there is changed or extraordinary in the patient. He writes all this down in the very words which the latter and the persons around him make use of. He permits them to continue speaking to the end without interruption, except where they wander into useless digressions, taking care to exhort them at the commencement to speak slowly that he may be enabled to follow them in taking down whatever he deems necessary.

One of the most important things in securing the image of a sickness is to preserve in simplicity what the patient tells us in his own way unless he digresses from the important things and talks about things that are foolish and not to the point; but as long as he confines his information to his own sufferings, let him tell it in his own way without interruption and in the record use his own language, only correcting his grammatical errors for the purpose of procuring the record as perfect as possible. If you use synonyms be sure that they are synonyms and cannot be perverted. Of course, when the woman speaks of her menstrual period as "monthlies" or as her "show," the more suitable medical term is "menses," which is a synonym for those expressions, and is more expressive than her own way of calling it "a show". So in general terms you can substitute terms of expression so long as you do not change the idea. Of course, the changing of "legs" into "limbs" if you feel like making such a change is not a change of thought, but be sure in making a change it is not a change of thought.

It is one of the most important things in forming the record of a patient to be able to read it at a subsequent examination, wihout being disturbed by the repeated statements of the patient. If you write a record in consecutive sentences, you will be so confused when hunting out the symptoms of the patient that you will be unable to form an image of that sickness in the mind. It is truly impossible when the mind is full with the effort at hunting out something to listen with proper and concentrated attention. You should divide your page in such a manner that when the patient is talking to you about this thing and that thing and the other thing of her symptoms, you can with one glance of the eye look down over the page of the record and see everything there is in that page. If your record is not so arranged, it is defective. Now, a record can be so arranged by dividing the page into three columns, the first of which contains the dates and prescriptions, the second the emphatic symptoms or headings and the third things predicated of the symptoms, thus:

Date

Symptom.
    Things predicated of the symptom
    < (aggravation),
Remedy   > (amelioration).

After the patient has detailed his sufferings in his own way and you have gone through them and discovered all the things that you can predicate of his symptoms then you can proceed to make enquiry of some one who has been with this patient. In a study like this with most of our private patients there has been a nurse, sometimes only a sister or a mother or a wife, who has been observing all the sick individual has complained of. "The persons who are about him relate what he has complained of, how he has behaved himself, and all that they have remarked in him." Now, this should be listened to with great care. It is more important in this instance to decide whether the observer is overanxious, if a wife whether she is not frightened concerning her husband and so intermingles many of her notions and fears, which you must accept with discretion. Get the nurse, if possible, to repeat the exact words of the patient. If such a thing can be done in acute sufferings it is worth more than the words or expressions of the nurse, the wife for instance, because the more interested and anxious the person is the less likely she will be to present a truthful image, not that she wants to deceive, but she is dreadfully wrought up and the more she thinks of what he has said the greater his sufferings appear to her, and she exaggerates them. It is important to have the statement from one who is disinterested. Two or three of the observers who are intelligent having been consulted and their statements recorded, the physician then notes his own observations. He should describe the urine if there is anything peculiar about that, but if the urine and stool are normal he need not care about the description of these.

It has been the study for hundreds of years to find the best way to question witnesses in court, and as a result they have settled upon certain rules for obtaining evidence. Homœopathy also has rules for examining the case that must be followed with exactitude through private practice. Among pupils who have been taught here, I know some who have merely memorized and some have not even memorized but have fallen away. These students are violating everything they have been taught; they have gone to low potencies, making greater and greater failures, to the shame of the tutor and the science they profess to follow. I expect some in the sound of my voice will be doing this five years from now; this is a warning, stop before you go too far, or you will not feel the fault is your own. You will think you were hypnotized and led into false ways. If you neglect making a careful examination the patient will be the first sufferer, but in the end you yourself will suffer from it, and Homœopathy also. The questions themselves that Hahnemann gives are not important, but they are suggestive and will lead you in a certain direction. Question the patient, then the friends, and observe for yourself; if you do not obtain enough to prescribe on, go back to particulars. After much experience you will become expert in questioning patients so as to bring out the truth. Store up Materia Medica so as to use it and it will flow out as your language flows. You must put yourself on a level with the form of speech your patients use.

Be sure you have not put any words into your patient's mouth or biased his expression. You want to know all the particulars but without asking about it directly. If you ask a direct question, you must not put the symptom in the record, for ninety-nine times out of a hundred the patient will answer by 'Yes' or 'No.' If the patient's answer is 'Yes' or 'No,' your question was badly formed. If a question brings no answer let it alone, for he does not know or has not noticed. Questions giving a choice of answers are defective. Ascertain the precise part of the body the pain was in and the character of the pain, etc. In investigating a case there are many things to learn, the length of the attack, appearance of the discharge if it be a case of vomiting, its charater, the time of day, etc., etc. Every student should go over these questions framing collateral questions, and practising case-taking. Leave the patient in freedom always.

Do not put any words into his mouth. Never allow yourself to hurry a patient; get into a fixed habit of examination, then it will stay with you. It is only when you sustain the sharpest kind of work that you can keep your reputation and fulfil your highest use. Say as little as you can, but keep the patient talking and keep him talking close to the line. If he will only talk, you can find out symptoms in general and particular. If he goes off, bring him back to the line quietly and without disturbing him. There is not much trouble in private practice. There you will do a better average of work.

All sleep symptoms are important, they are so closely related to the mind, the transfer from sleep to waking, from cerebrum to cerebellum, is important. Old pathologists were unable to account for difficult breathing during sleep. The cerebrum rules respiration during sleep. To know the functions of the white matter and gray matter is important. A rational knowledge of anatomy is important. No homœopath ever discouraged the true study of anatomy and physiology. It is important not only to know the superficial but the real, profound character, to enable you to recognize one symptom-image from another.

Study this paragraph carefully and meditate upon it. If you do not form habits now, you will not form practice hereafter. You have no regular course and will get into habits you cannot break up.

LECTURE XXIV

THE EXAMINATION OF THE PATIENT (*Continued*)

The examination must be continued with due respect to the nature of the sickness and with due respect to the nature of the Materia Medica. Some symptoms have reference to pathology and diagnosis, while others have reference only to the Materia Medica, and symptoms must be constantly weighed in the mind in order to establish their grade whether common or peculiar. If all are found to be common symptoms, the Materia Medica is left out. Either the examination has not been made with respect to the Materia Medica, or the symptoms are not there at all. It makes no difference as far as cure is concerned; it matters not whether they are not present in the case or whether the doctor has not found them, the key to the prescription is not present. But if the image is round and full and complete, there are symptoms with regard to pathology, diagnosis, prognosis and Materia Medica. It will be proper later to talk of incurable diseases, pathognomic symptoms, obscure cases, Materia Medica symptoms, etc.

When the physician comes to look over the record after an examination to get the image to classify and arrange it, he will find what is peculiar, and those symptoms that are most general, and those that are but common. These three grades appear in every complete case, and in every complete proving of a remedy. Homœopathic study and observation will enable one to pick out these grades at a glance. Every case has common symptoms, but peculiar symptoms may be absent and you must not expect to cure when peculiar symptoms are absent. Homœopathy is applicable in every curable case, but the great thing is to know how to apply it. The physician must sit in judgment upon the symptoms and determine whether they are peculiar or common. If the patient's discourse is incoherent, the question arises is he intoxicated or delirious, or is there breaking down of the brain and insanity? The flash of the eye is important; it will tell things that cannot be told by the nurse.

It is important for the physician to know the value of expressions. When the patient stares with glassy eye, is he injured about the head, is he suffering from shock, intoxication or typhoid fever, or some disease in which the mind is stunned? The physician immediately proceeds to ask, "How long has the patient been in bed?" If the character is above reproach, he will not suspect intoxication; if the patient has been sick for many days with fever, tongue coated, abdomen sensitive, etc., he is fully entered upon the course of typhoid fever. The physician must know immediately upon entering the room what the state of the patient resembles: apoplexy, coma, opium poisoning, etc. A physician is supposed to set his mind to work instantly, to ascertain the condition of the patient and what relation the symptoms maintain to the Materia Medica. If an opium poisoning there must be selected an antidote; if apoplexy, a careful taking of the symptoms in relation to the cerebral clot to prevent inflammation and symptoms relative to that state, and relative to the remedy. The patient may be intoxicated and have apoplexy at the same time. There is no symptom in the sick room without its value, especially in acute and serious cases. Children are sometimes found in a sound sleep and cannot be aroused; the mother says the child has worms and gives Cina, for Cina has all these symptoms of stupor, difficulty in arousing, falling back to sleep. But the child fails, going into coma, the nose flaps, the chest heaves, the brow is wrinkled, there is rattling in the chest, showing the child is going into cerebral congestion. The physician now must examine on every side of the case to find the nature, to know what to expect. He who neglects this is not a true homœopathic physician; a mere superficial application of Homœopathy is not sufficient. After all the symptoms are written out, the physician must study the character of the fever, whether it is intermittent, continued or has come on in one sudden attack; he must know sufficient of the symptoms to judge of all these. You will learn so much about the purport and the aspect of every motion of the human being that you will place less and less reliance on diagnostic symptoms as diagnostic symptoms, and learn more the value of symptoms as symptoms. You will be astonished to find how expert you will become about diagnosis and prognosis by studying the symptoms. You can learn something from every case you have mind; but by a process of rapid exclusion, you say it is not into mind; but by a process of rapid exclusion, you say it is not cholera, not hemorrhage, etc., and latterly you come to the cause of this aspect. You can tell when it is time for cardiac compensation to be broken in Bright's disease; a peculiar tremulous wave that belongs to the muscles of the face and neck, a tremulous jerk of the tongue, putting about half way; the pale, cold, semi-transparent skin with cold sweat. It is important to know instantly what the cause is, for the treatment will be different, but remember that it is nothing that you need to name that makes it important.

All these symptoms have respect to remedy and to diagnostic conditions. So far as there is a morbid anatomy which can account for symptoms, so much less are those symptoms worth, as indicating a remedy; if you had no other than such symptoms, you could find no remedy.

Among the many things that interfere with the examination of the patient the most important is the taking of medicines, or having done something, no matter what it is, that has been capable of changing the symptoms. Very commonly, the patient will present himself in the doctor's office, and after giving a long array of symptoms will relate a dose of Quinine, and he thinks he is no better, and now he applies to you for relief. In acute diseases this is very bad and may interfere with finding the homœopathic remedy. Very often the general state collectively both drug and disease symptoms, in a very acute condition must be prescribed for, but in chronic disease the plan is different. The symptoms that arise after the taking of a dose of powerful medicine are not indicative of a remedy, they are confusing, they present no true image of the disease and hence the physician has nothing to do but wait, or at most administer a well-known antidote to the drug taken. Sometimes he must wait a considerable time until the symptoms reveal themselves and express the nature of the sickness. It is just as bad where the physician himself is a bungler as it is where the patient has taken the drugs. The confusion arising from bad prescribing is just the same as that produced by the patient's drugging. There are physicians going about who will mix up their cases and continue to prescribe for their own drug symptoms, and who never have any idea of waiting for the true image of the disease to develop itself. Drugging is only a matter of changing symptoms and masking the case. Anything that will effect a change in the symptoms, the taking of drugs, or drinking too much wine or drinking toddy, or great exposure, will mask the case, and this mask must wear away before the intelligent physician can make a cure. The whole aim of the physician is to secure the language of nature. If it has been masked by medicines, it cannot be secured. Any meddling will so affect the aspect of the case that the physician cannot prescribe, and the physician who does this meddling must inevitably be driven into bad methods or into allopathy. I have looked over the work of bad prescribers and have wondered what on earth they could see in Homœopathy to attract them; they do not cure folks. They have no cures to present. The patients cannot well be satisfied by these things. It is true that once in a while a strong, vigorous, robust patient, when he gets a homœopathic remedy, will go on getting well through a mess of symptom changing and drugging, so that in spite of this meddlesome practice he will recover. The physician in that case, knows not what remedy to attribute to it, for he has given a great many. But only the most vigorous constitution will stand such homœopathic villainy, go on and get well in spite of their indulgence in wine, in eating, etc.; it is wonderful what their own powers will do in throwing off disease.

In ordinary cases, however, we see no such things; confusion is brought about at once if the physician administer another medicine in place of administering placebo. At times a patient will present himself, and you will be able to get a true image of the sickness by ascertaining all the things that occurred up to a given date. "Upon that date," he says, "I took some medicine, and most of my symptoms subsided." They lead to another image from which you can gather nothing; a scattering has taken place. The symptoms may cover page upon page, and yet what remedy do you see? None at all; it looks as if a number of provings of drugs had been mixed up all together, intermingling symptoms here and there without any distinctness. No individualization is possible. Now up to that date the symptoms you gathered may be just all that is necessary. Up to that date the symptoms present the image of a remedy which, if administered, may yet act, though sometimes it will fail at first because of the confusion, but after waiting a little it will act. After the administration of a remedy prescribed upon symptoms in the past I have known the remedy many times to go on acting. Again I have known that remedy to fail entirely. In such a case, wait awhile and then order will begin to come and that remedy which was indicated previous to the drugging will act. Suppose a physician comes to you and says, "Up to a certain date I was able to hold this patient's symptoms in order with Thuja; but then the symptoms seemed to change and I gave such and such medicines, and have never seen such good results in prescribing as I did up to that period." You must give him Thuja again, and in this way take up the thread where it was lost. Examine the image of the case where the order was lost; because that is where the image must be found. "On the contrary, the symptoms and the inconveniences which exhibited themselves previous to the use of the medicines, or several days after their discontinuance, give the true fundamental notion of the original form of the malady."

This is the idea, get the original form of the malady. To do this, at times we have to trace through a mass of difficulties and conditions to get back to the original form of the trouble, but you must get there because you will see that in the beginning this malady, in accordance with all laws of Divine Providence, must have conformed to some remedy that had been created for its cure. The symptoms at that time stood out indicating this medicine, but since then there has been nothing but confusion, nothing that can be tied to, nothing that can be examined; it appears to have no relation to anything. Very often we can take up the thread and get back to the remedy that was clearly indicated, even twenty years before. If that remedy was indicated then, and was not given, the cure that was possible by that remedy or a similar one is the only thing to be considered; that is the only remedy in the case. Since that time the patient has been in continued turmoil from the action of drugs. Because it was twenty years ago there is no reason that you should not think of that drug. The patient's disease has not been cured, it has only been changed and modified; but it is the same patient, and the same sickness and requires the same medicine. If the disease has been complicated by drugs, however, you cannot always get the action of that medicine which the patient needs for the disease *per se*, but after the drugs have been antidoted you will have to give that very medicine that you figured out and he will be cured.

It is necessary also to observe the changes all along the line of progress, to know the disease at its beginnings, its earlier manifestations, its symptoms and its endings. You find, say, most violent neuralgic pains along the course of nerves in an adult patient, and for these you administer remedies until you are tired and get only temporary relief; but you discover that in his childhood he had an eczema, and you will find it looks like Mezereum, and see its violent neuralgias are similar to those of your patient. The administration of Mezereum cures this neuralgia and brings back the eruption that he had in his babyhood, and he goes on to recovery. Without getting that view of the old scald head, you would not have thought of Mezereum.

Or, instead of Mezereum, Sepia may have had the likeness of that scald head, and he may now have the most striking and characteristic symptoms of Sepia; for behold the little things that have been put into such a turmoil by a bad drugging are under Sepia, and you put your patient on Sepia, and these last appearing symptoms go first and the eruption comes back upon the head and behind the ears, and Sepia has cured him. When these things are seen one after another in everyday practice the physician must begin to wonder if there is not some truth in it all. And as sure as you live, if you practice faithfully, carefully studying your cases at great length, gathering in everything that was in the beginning, your cures will be so striking that the multitude will come to you to be healed. You cannot place too much importance upon the masking of a patient's symptoms by medicines, by improper repetitions and by dosing carelessly.

§ 94. "On inquiry into a state of chronic disease it is required to weigh the particular circumstances in which the patient may be placed in regard to ordinary occupation, mode of life and domestic situation," etc. Almost everything in life is circumstantial. All of the activities of life are circumstantial, i.e., there are no activities that are not governed by circumstance. There is no business that is not governed by circumstance. The circumstances of a man's life govern his actions and reactions, symptoms and the development of symptoms. The body is associated with circumstances, every function is related to circumstance, and we may say all the natural functions of life are connected with circumstances. Without these we would have nothing to prescribe upon, we would have nothing to ascertain images by, we would have nothing to form the symptoms, hence the circumstances of life and habit must be studied with a view to going into the slightest particulars. To illustrate that more particularly, and to bring it down to a practical basis, we may say that the examination of every woman relates to her eating, her stool, her menstruation, her bathing, her dress, because these are the things natural to her. These are the circumstances in which her symptoms may come or may not come.

Until the woman is educated to it she does not understand.

"What do you mean, Doctor?" she says. Then I may say, "You have given me these symptoms; you say you have headache, stomachache, etc. Now will you proceed to relate to me under what circumstances this headache appears, how it is affected by your changes in dress, by the changes in weather, how it is affected before, during or after your monthly indisposition and so on." Now, these are the natural circumstances.

In addition to these another group of circumstances comes up, a group of circumstances somewhat different, in relation to ordinary occupation. Every person will have circumstances more particular than those in general. Occupation will make changes in the circumstances of young women. She may be standing upon the floor of Wanamaker's store all day, and this has produced a condition of prolapsus; or she may lead a sedentary life at her work as seamstress, or she may be at some other occupation, the circumstance of which will develop her psoric manifestations. Modes of life mean a great many different things. They come in as supernumeraries over and above the natural conditions and circumstances of life. The natural functions and circumstances of life have to be considered in relation to the mode of life. The mode of life comes in as the exciting cause of disease, whereby psora which is in the economy is developed in a certain peculiar direction.

The domestic is often the cause of trouble in the woman; there may be marriage to a man who is intemperate with her sexually; she may have a domestic situation that cannot be cured, and it must be examined as to its permanency and the prospect of removing it. Things that cannot be removed will develop psora, in a peculiar direction. "All these circumstances ought to be examined to discover if there is anything that could give birth to and keep up the disease, so that by its removal the cure may be facilitated."

LECTURE XXV

THE EXAMINATION OF THE PATIENT (Continued)

§ 92. The patients generally call attention to the commonest things, while it is the strange and peculiar things that guide to a remedy. The symptoms most covered up from the observation of the physician are often the things guiding to the remedy, but finally they leak out in some way. The symptom is of such a character that the patient says of it, "I have always had it and did not suppose that had anything to do with my disease." When asked, "Why did you not tell me that before?" she says, "I did not suppose that amounted to anything, it is so trivial." The physician often hazards a remedy. He feels he must make a prescription, but has no reasonable grounds for thinking he has found the remedy because the patient's story has been so confusing, and the symptoms that he has obtained are so common and ordinary, such as all remedies possess. With such a foundation he cannot have any assurance that he has the remedy, and, although he may have hazarded several remedies in the case, the patient comes back uncared, month after month, and year after year. These symptoms that are withheld and seem to be so obscure, and so difficult to obtain, are the very ones that the patient thinks do not amount to anything. What seems to him to be the little symptoms are very often characteristic of the disease, and necessary for the choice of the remedy. Let me illustrate it. A patient comes along with a pallid face, a rather sickly countenance, tired and weary, subject to headaches, disorders of the bladder and disturbances of digestion; and in spite of all your questioning, you fail to get anything that is peculiar. You set the patient to thinking and to writing down symptoms, and she comes back month after month and give her *Sulphur, Lycopodium* and a good many medicines. You can sometimes find out whether she is a chilly or hot-blooded patient, and thus you can get a little closer among the common remedies; but the patient says one day, "Doctor, it seems strange that urine smells so queer, it smells like that of a horse." Now at once you know that is *Nitric acid*. "How long have you had this?" "Oh, I have always had it, I did not think it amounted to anything." If you examine the common things belonging to *Nitric acid* you will find that it possesses all the features of the case.

This is how a guiding symptom can be used. *Nitric acid* has a keynote "urine smelling strong like that of a horse;" but if you should give it upon that alone and the general symptoms were not there, you would probably remove the particular symptoms only, and they would come back after a while. Use a keynote to examine the remedy to see if it has all the other symptoms that the patient has. What I have described to you is a hypothetical case. In a busy day you will have several of these cases that you have been working at for months, and the patients have spent a lot of money to no account. You might just as well have given *Sac. lac.* until you found the right remedy. You can hardly say, why did I not see the remedy before, because it was not possible to see it. You can only go over a case and say, why did I not ask her if there was any odor to the urine, and if so, what it was like. I have had this very symptom come out when I have asked a dozen times about the smell of the urine, and they did not know, and yet would say afterwards their urine smelled like a horse's urine, and they knew it all the time. "On the other hand, the patients are so accustomed to their long sufferings that they pay little or no attention to the lesser symptoms which are often characteristic of the disease and decisive in regard to the choice of a remedy."

Of course the trouble that we have to contend with in ascertaining symptoms from patients could be drawn out to great length. You might suppose that it would be the educated class that would tell their symptoms best, but you will find the ignorant class often do better, they are simpler; they do not disguise the symptoms; they come out and tell the little details in a better way, in a way that conforms to the language of our remedies. Our remedies have been recorded in simple language to a great extent, and this simple language is often better observed by the simple-minded, uncultivated people than among the aristocrats. People who have plenty of means and much education are more excitable, they have more fear and they have tried a great many doctors. Any physician who has a reputation is consulted for a chronic disease; and the patient who has plenty of money goes around amongst the doctors, and when he comes to tell his symptoms he tells them in the technicalities of his numerous physicians, so that when he has finished his story nothing has been gained. Only gradually can the physician lead him back into a language simple enough to describe the sufferings. They who have been sick long with their chronic ailments and have become somewhat hypochondriac will go through with this list of their diseases. They have paid lots of money, and have lots of names, and they are loaded with drugs. The physician must deal very carefully with these slippery people, because if they are irritated they will run off.

§ 96. There is another kind of patient spoken of here, those that "depict their sufferings in lively colors, and make use of exaggerated terms to induce the physician to relieve them promptly. This is especally characteristc of the native Irish as a class. You will find that they will exaggerate their symptoms, really and sincerely believing that tho doctor will give them stronger medicine if they are very sick and will pay more attention to them; and if they do not exaggerate violently, probably he will turn them off with a simple remedy. Then we have the exaggeration of symptoms by sensitive people. It is an insane habit, such as belong to hysteria. The physician will be helpless in the hands of these exaggerators, because Homœopathy consists in securing the whole truth and nothing but the truth; it is just as detrimental to get too much as to get too little. Any coloring that is expressed, whether by the patient or by the physician, will result in failure. It is true that this tendency to exaggeration must be considered as a symptom. When you have found a patient to exaggerate a few symptoms into a large number, you can simply mention in your note "tendency to exaggerate symptoms," which is covered by some of our remedies. Such a state is misleading, for you do not know what symptoms the patient has and what the patient has not. You may rest assured that no patient without symptoms would consult a physiciain; the patient would not be likely to manufacture the entire sickness; the fact that she has a desire to present herself to the physician and has a desire to exaggerate her symptoms and sufferings is in itself a disease, because no well person would do that. Hence this must be considered; perhaps it is the first and only element that can be considered of that which such patients give out. This exaggeration must be measured with discretion and wisdom. "Even the most impatient hypochrondriac never invents sufferings and symptoms that are void of foundation, and the truth of this is easily ascertained by comparing the complaints he utters at different intervals while the physician gives him nothing at least that is medicinal." Hahnemann's plan would be to give no medicine and to compare the symptoms that the patient gives from time to time. The patient cannot memorize these various symptoms that he has gathered from other sources, but by watching and comparing from time to time, letting the examination be far enough apart for him to forget, the physician can accept those things that he repeats. The young physician will be misguided by these cases until he has had sufficient experience with disease to know something about the nature of symptoms that ought to appear.

Another obstacle we have in the examination of the case is laziness; the patient is too lazy to write down the symptoms when they appear, and too indolent and forgetful to remember them in the presence of the physician. The symptoms do not come up in his mind when he is in the presence of the doctor, and he is too indolent to write these symptoms down when he feels them at home. When a patient does not relate symptoms well he should be instructed to write down his symptoms when they occur, and if he will not do that his physician should insist upon it, or refuse to prescribe for him. It is often quite an important thing to get the patient to write down the symptoms in memorandum form as they occur. Not to write at night what has occurred during the day, but to run instantly and put the symptom down in simple language, describing the sensation, and location, and the time of day of its coming and going, and the modalities. Indolence then and forgetfulness become obstacles to the gathering of the symptoms.

Now, in the present day, there has crept upon the face of the earth such a state of false modesty and such a lack of innocence upon the whole human race that this false modesty and shame will prevent patients from telling the truth. Patients will deny having had gonorrhœa, or having been exposed to circumstances that were similar. If the whole human race had lived in innocence up to the present day our women would come to the physician with frankness and talk in perfect freedom concerning the menstrual flow, concerning even the sexual functions, concerning things of the will and of the intelligence. But as a matter of fact it is not so, it is with difficulty that the physicians can draw out these symptoms through mistaken modesty. When a patient consults a physician, the question of modesty should be laid aside. You will find that the most innocent in mind are those that are the most easy to lay it aside, when it is not a question of modesty, but of telling the whole truth and nothing but the truth. If it be a wife, everything that is in relation to herself and husband that is abnormal should be told, and then the physician would have little to ask beyond listening to the truth. I look back over a number of people, especially among women, when seemed to be so much embarrassed upon first coming into my presence and having to talk about their symptoms that they forget everything, and it was only by considerable waiting that they became free and frank and open with me. Sometimes it is a difficult matter for the physician to put a patient at ease; it is a thing that must be studied and considered in order to be able to say something to put a bashful patient at ease; this is quite an accomplishment with a doctor.

The physician must be possessed of an uncommon share of circumspection and tact, a knowledge of the human heart, prudence and patience, to be enabled to form to himself a true and complete image of the disease in all its details. He must live the life of the neighbor, and be known as a man of honor, as a man who may be believed and respected, as a candid man. Hahnemann says carelessness, laziness and levity will prevent the physician from going into such a state of Homœopathy as will enable him to grasp the Materia Medica or to be conversant with his science. If he has such a reputation he will not command the respect of the people of the neighborhood, and this will prevent him from getting the image of the sickness upon paper. Hahnemann had a wonderful knowledge of the human heart, and this is an important thing; a knowledge of the human heart, a knowledge of the things that are in man.

It would seem that there are a good many men in the community without the slightest knowledge of the human heart. They have never given any inspection to their own interiors, their heart or impulses, but have gone on wildly. To know the human heart well is largely to examine into oneself and ascertain what one's own impulses are, what one is compelled to do under varying circumstances, what impulses one has to control in oneself in order to become a man. If a man has carried out his heart's desires without any self-control he is a man unworthy of respect. If he has on the other hand controlled those impulses, he has become a man worthy of respect. In time the physician who does this will become so well acquainted with the human heart that he has sympathy and knows what constitutes the language of the affections.

LECTURE XXVI

THE EXAMINATION OF THE PATIENT (*Continued*)

It is important to avoid getting confused by two disease images that may exist in the body at the same time. A chronic patient, for instance, may be suffering from an acute disease and the physician on being called may think that it is necessary to take the totality of the symptoms; but if he should do that in an acute disease, mixing both chronic and acute symptoms together, he will become confused and will not find the right remedy. The two things must be separated. The group of symptoms that constitutes the image and appearance of the acute miasm must now be prescribed for. The chronic symptoms will not, of course, be present when the acute miasm is running, because the latter suppresses or suspends the chrronic symptoms, but the diligent physician, not knowing this is so, might wrongly gather together all the symptoms that the patient has had in a life time. Again, on the other hand, in gathering together the chronic symptoms for a prescription it is sufficient to mention merely that the patient has had typhoid or measles or other actute miasms. Such diseases are not a part of the chronic miasm. The symptoms of the acute attack were separate and by themselves.

You must realize that the effort to prescribe for two distinct miasms will result in error. If you practice in the western part of this country you will often get confused cases, a sample of which would be about as follows: A patient has been suffering from intermittent fever, and has been treated with medicines, Quinine, Arsenic and low potencies of this and that drug, until the case has been complicated. You learn that the symptoms now are different from what they were in the beginning, that there has been a transformation scene. You prescribe for them as they are now, regarding it as a species of malaria; you prescribe for them with a view to antidoting all the drugs that he has had, and your remedy brings about a surprise; it opens out the case in a wonderful manner. The patient up to this time was unable to give you anything descriptive of the original state of his malaria, but he comes back in the course of a week or two and says: "Doctor, I am now as I was in the beginning." "Well, what are your symptoms now?" And you will find out that one evening he has a 5 o'clock chill with its accompanying symptoms that last him a good portion of the night, and then he has a well day, and then next forenoon he has an 11 o'clock chill and then a well day. If you examine each one of these states, you will find that the two chills begin in a different place, and the heat of each begins in a different place, and the symptoms of the two attacks are totally different. Such a thing will seem unlikely to one who has never seen it, but one who has lived in the west and practiced accurately will see such things, unknown to those who have practiced what is called Quinine Homœopathy. A correct prescription will disentangle these two malarial miasms and show that two exist in the body at the same time, each having conditions quite different from the other. These two can co-exist and have their own times and expressions without interfering with each other to any great extent. The big doses of quinine will complicate them and cause a general clouding of things, so helter-skelter and disorderly that nobody can tell anything about it.

If in such a case you were to attempt to prescribe a remedy that had both these groups you would fail to cure. Select the worst one, and let the other one alone, entirely ignoring it. It is a bad policy to give one remedy for one and another for the other. Single out the worst one and cover it carefully with a remedy, and you will find it disappear and the other one comes on, just as if the patient had not a remedy at all.

Now do not be in too great a hurry about removing the second one. You will find that after one has been removed the patient will improve, and the one that has remained will become more and more apparent from day to day; then prescribe for it.

This illustrates the doctrine of not prescribing for an acute and chronic trouble together. Never prescribe for any two conditions, unless they be complicated. Only chronic diseases can be complicated with each other. The acute is never complicated with the chronic; the acute suppresses the chronic and they never become complex. Of course, the allopaths will tell you about the sequelæ of measles, scarlet fever, etc., but they know nothing about it, and their pathology teaches them nothing which is true concerning it. That which comes out after all self-limiting diseases have run their course is not due to the disease itself; the sequelæ of measles are not due to measles, the sequelæ of scarlet fever are not due to scarlet fever, but to a prior state of the patient. A psoric disorder may come after scarlet fever or measles, and must be treated as psora.

These sequelæ, regardless of the disease which stirs them up, are psoric and crop out at the weakest time, which is the convalescent period. The better the acute disease is treated, the less likely there are to be any sequelæ. If measles and scarlet fever are treated properly we have very little trouble afterwards. Sequelæ should always be charged up to a great extent to the physician. Of course, you will find now and then some constitutions extremely psoric; almost in a condition of advanced decay, and for malignant scarlet fever in such a patient it is difficult to find a proper remedy, and then the very best physician in the world may make a mistake; yet with good treatment in ordinary cases you should not expect sequelæ, such as sore eyes, running ears, etc.

It is of the greatest importance in such cases to be able to separate and distinguish one thing from another, so that you may know what you are prescribing for. You cannot prescribe an antipsoric in order to prevent sequelæ following scarlet fever while the scarlet fever prevails. Prescribe first for the acute attack, and the symptoms that belong to it. It is well, however, for the physician to know all the symptoms that the patient has of a chronic character, that he may know what to expect, that he may look at the close of the acute attack for the coming out of the old manifestations of psora, although often an entirely new group of symptoms will appear. When at the close of scarlet fever troubles come about the ears or dropsical conditions come on; these are not a part of the scarlet fever itself, but of the state of the economy. The dropsical condition, or acute Bright's disease, must be associated with the psoric state and the symptoms then will lead you to a constitutional remedy. If you have in view simply the Bright's disease, you will make a mistake. You will fall into prescribing for ultimates if you have but the name of the trouble in mind, for instance giving Apis, which the books say, is a wonderful remedy for Bright's disease, following scarlet fever.

It is a great mistake for anyone to fit remedies for complaints or states. It is a fatal error for the physician to go on the bedside of a patient with the feeling in his mind that he has had cases similar to this one, and thinking thus: "In the last case I had I gave so and so, therefore I will give it to this one." The physician must get such things entirely out of his mind. It is a common feature among occulists who profess to be homœopaths to say: "I cured such and such a case with such and such a remedy. I will now give this patient the same remedy." I have many times met physicians in consultations who said: "I have another patient, Mr. Z or Mr. X, who had a similar state of affairs, just such a disease as this, and I gave him so and so, but it does not work in this case."

§ 100. "With regard to a search after the totality of the symptoms in epidemic and sporadic cases, it is wholly indifferent whether anything similar ever existed before in the world or not, under any name whatever." Keep that in your mind, underscore it half a dozen times with red ink, paint it on the wall, put an index finger to it. One of the most important things is to keep out of the mind, in an examination of the case, some other case that has appeared to be similar. If this is not done the mind will be prejudiced in spite of your best endeavors. I have to fight that with every fresh case I come to. I have to labour to keep myself from thinking about things I have cured like that before, because it would prejudice my mind.

The purpose of all this is that you will go away and examine the patient with an unprejudiced mind, that you will consider only the case before you, that you will have nothing in mind that will distract your attention, that you may not think of things that preceded it and find out from among them a remedy while examining the patient. If you are biased in your judgment and examine the patient towards a certain remedy, in many instances this will prove to be fatal. Have no remedy in mind until you have everything that you can get on paper. Have it all written down carefully and then if, upon examining it in relation to remedies, you are unable to distinguish between three or four, you can go back and re-examine the patient with reference to those three or four remedies.

That is the only possible time you try to fit a remedy, or image of a remedy, while examining a patient. Get all the symptoms first and then commence your analysis in relation to remedies. The analysis of a sickness is for the purpose of gathering together that about it which is peculiar, for the peculiar thing relate to remedies. Sicknesses have in them that which is peculiar, strange and rare, and the things in sickness that may be wondererd at are things to be compared with those in the remedy that are peculiar. Now in order to see that which is wonderful and strange it is necessary for you to have much knowledge of disease and much knowledge of Materia Medica; not so much an extensive knowledge of morbid anatomy, but a knowledge of the symptoms or the language that disease expresses itself in. "In fact, we ought to regard the pure image of each prevailing disease as a thing that is new and unknown, and study the same from its foundation, if we would really exercise the art of healing." A great deal depends upon a physician's ability to perceive what constitutes the miasm. If he is dull of perception he will intermingle symptoms that do not belong together. Hahnemann seems to have had the most wonderful perception, he seemed to see at a glance. Hahnemann was skilful in this respect because he was a hard student of Materia Medica and because he proved his Materia Medica daily. He had examined the remedies carefully, he saw them, he felt them, he realized them. "We ought never to substitute hypothesis in the room of observation, never regard any case as already known." Now we see why it is that it does not make any difference with a physician whether he has seen such diseases before or not. The homœopathic physician is acquainted with the signs and symptoms of the man, and a different disease is only a change in the combination of them, only a change in their manner, form and representation. There is order, perfect order, in every sickness that presents itself, and it rests with the physician to find that order. The homœopathic physician need never be taken unawares.

LECTURE XXVII

RECORD KEEPING

§ 103, ETC.

You should endeavor to have a good knowledge of both the acute and chronic miasms. First of all the image of psora should be studied from all the symptoms that we can gather, and especially from the symptoms that Hahnemann has given, in the *Chronic Diseases*. Next we have to make out a similar anamnesis of syphilis, which can be done from books, from clinics, from observation, and all other possible sources, and then an anamnesis has to be made of sycosis. These are things most general, and will bring before the mind, in one, two or three images, a grand picture of all the chronic diseases of the human race.

Take psora first for that is the very foundation of human sickness. It would appear that the human race is one enormous leper. Now, add to that the state of syphilis and we have a bad matter made worse; then add to that the state of sycosis and we will see the extent of human sickness.

We then have to advance and carefully study each of the acute miasms from the books, from observation, and from every source of information, carefully arranging it on paper so that it can appear before the mind as an image. Smallpox has few features and it can be made to appear as an image before the mind, and so with all the acute miasms, infectious diseases, cholera, yellow fever, etc., the diseases that have heretobefore appeared in epidemic or endemic form. These have all to appear before the mind as images. It may be said of them that they are all true diseases seen by the examination of the totality of the symptoms. No physician can know too much about the image of a given sickness, studied from the symptomatology, and this is the best information that can be obtained. Now-a-days patients are not permitted to tell their story in the language of nature. The physician says, "I do not want to hear that." Talk on the part of the patient interferes with his prescription writing. There is no writing down of the case.

Now take, for instance, one of the clinics here. How would you remember from day to day, and from week to week, what had been given to each patient? There is no importance attached to that in the old school. It is simply their object to give the patient a big dose of medicine. It may not have occurred to you that there are several reasons of importance for keeping records, and of constantly referring to them; even the regular clinicians here may not have seen the full importance of it. But suppose a patient that I have been considering for three years is partially cured, and she has done remarkably well, has been restored from an invalid to a good wife and mother, but is not yet cured. Now for some reason she goes into the hands of another homœopath. What can he do without ascertaining what I have done for her? It is important for the patient when living in the same town to be faithful and true to the physician who has done her the most good. A conscientious physician will not feel like taking another doctor's practice in that way. I am not so conceited that I should feel like taking up the work of another doctor who is able to do good work. Men who think more of getting money than anything else will jump in and prescribe for your patients.

"The physician ought ever after to have this image before the eyes to serve as a basis to the treatment, especially where the disease is chronic." Without records, you are at sea without compass or rudder. With a record, Hahnemann says, "He can then study it in all its parts, and draw from it the characteristic marks," that is, you have the nature of the disease continuously in mind. When the image of the disease has passed from mind its very nature is gone.

Here a point comes in you must know about. After your first prescription has been made, you may have an aggravation. It is well to know the date of this, and about how long it lasted, and to keep watch of it. If no change has occurred the same image may continue to appear before the mind, but if changes have occurred and are continuously appearing in the symptoms you will readily see that no medicine can be administered. The symptoms that come and go could not guide anybody as to what to do. Now a commotion has taken place, you cannot prescribe while this commotion is going on, the symptoms are changing place, they are coming and going, for perhaps one to three weeks after that prescription. You have to watch and wait. Notice when the symptoms begin to roll into order; then another dose of medicine is needed.

These things take place only after the administration of a remedy that was pretty high, high enough to take hold, and the case falls into order only when the patient needs another dose.

Suppose a patient has been sick three to four years with a train of symptoms, and on the way to visit you from a long distance; the patient is taken worse, and a homœopathic physician is called in. The patient gets a dose of medicine and improves wonderfully, now what are you going to do? You do not know what it was and you write to the physician, but he has forgotten what it was. What a confusing state that is, is it not? Well, that is just the state you would be in without your records.

There is, I have been led to feel, too great carelessness often among our best men in transferring cases from one town to another, from one physician to another. A habit that has existed between another Hahnemannian and myself has been pleasing to us both. When one of his patients has been transferred from his care to my care he has told me what remedy the patient was on, and I in the same way when sending patients to him have mentioned the remedy the patient was on. It is the duty of the physician to furnish such information when a patient leaves the city to go under the care of another physician. It is the duty of the physician to transfer such a patient to good hands, if there are any good hands to transfer him to.

This subject is preliminary to the observation of § 105, which leads to the second step of practical Homœopathy.

LECTURE XXVIII

THE STUDY OF PROVINGS

§ 105, *et. seq.*

It may be well for you to review thoroughly the first portion of the study of the *Organon*, containing the doctrines in general that may be hereafter found to be useful in the application of Homœopathy, including the oldest established rules and principles. The first step may be called theoretical Homœopathy, or the principles of Homœopathy after which we take up the homœopathic method of studying sickness. In this way we have found that the study of sickness in our school is entirely different from the study of sickness under the old school. But up to this time the doctrines have not exhibited their purpose; we only get their purpose when we come to the third step, which deals with the use of Materia Medica. We have seen that we must study sickness by gathering the symptoms of sick patients, relying upon the symptoms as the language of nature, and that the totality of the symptoms constitutes the nature and quality and all there is that is to be known of the disease.

The subject we will now take up and consider is, how to acquire a knowledge of the instruments that we shall make use of in combating human sickness. We know very well that in the old school there is no plan laid down for acquiring a knowledge of medicines except by experimenting with them upon the sick. This Hahnemann condemns as dangerous, because it subjects human sufferers to hardship and because of its uncertainty. Though this system has existed for many hundreds of years, it has never revealed a principle or method that one can take hold of to help in curing the sickness of the human family. His experiments in drug proving were made before he studied diseases. In other words, Hahnemann built the Materia Medica and then took up the plan of examining the patient to see what remedy the sickness looked like. Whereas now, after Homœopathy has been established, and the Materia Medica has been established, the examination of the patient precedes, in a particular case, the examination of the Materia Medica. But for the purpose of study they go hand in hand.

Before Hahnemann could examine the Materia Medica you may say he had to make one, for there was none to examine, there were no provings as yet; we now have the instruments before us to examine, we have the proved remedies. When the fallacy of old school medicine fully entered Hahnemann's mind; when he became disgusted with its method at the time his children were sick; when he placed himself in the stream of Providence and affirmed his trust that the Lord had not made these little ones to suffer, and then to be made worse from violent medicines; then his mind was in an attitude for discovery. It was a discountenancing of and disgust for the things that were useless, and this brought him to the state of acknowledgment of not knowing and that everything of man's own opinion must be thrown away. It brought him to a state of humility and the acknowledgment of Divine Providence.

The state of humility opens man's mind. You will find so long as man is in a position to trust himself he makes himself a god; he makes himself the infallible; he looks to himself and does not see beyond himself; his mind is then closed. When a man finds out that in himself he is a failure, that is the beginning of knowledge in any circumstance; the very opposite of this closes the mind and turns man away from knowledge.

I have been teaching long enough to observe, and I will tell you some things I have observed. I have observed quite a number of young people turn away from Homœopathy after once confessing it, and professing to practice it, and after seeming able in a certain degree to practice it. I often wondered why it was that after they had made public profession of it they turned away from it, and I found in every instance that it was due to lack of humility. The great mistake comes from turning one's attention into self and relying upon self, with an attention that closes the mind and deprives one of knowledge and prevents clear perception. Man takes himself out of the stream of Providence when he becomes dissatisfied with himself and thinks "now that I have done so many things I have nothing more to study." This is a wrong attitude; for anything like self-conceit will blind a man's eyes, will make him unable to use the means of cure and will prevent his becoming acquainted with the Materia Medica. The homœopathic physician, as much as the clergyman, ought to keep himself in a state of purity, a state of humility, a state of innocence. So sure as he does not do that he will fall by the wayside. There is nothing that destroys a man so fast in the scientific world as conceit. We see in old-fashioned science men who are puffed up and corpulent with conceit. The scientific men who are in the greatest degree of simplicity are the most wise and the most worthy, and you need not tell me that those who are innocent and simple have not had a tremendous struggle in order to keep self under control and to reach this state of simplicity.

Extensive knowledge makes a man simple, makes him gentle. Extensive knowledge makes a man realize how little he knows, and what a small concern he is. A little knowledge makes a fool of man, and makes him think he knows it all, and the more he forgets of what he has known the bigger man he feels he is. The smaller he feels he is the more he knows, you may rest assured. In order to do this, he must study and keep himself in a state of gravity and in a state of innocence.

In the scientific world we have all those horrible jealousies and feelings of hatred to those who know more than we do. A man who cannot control that and keep that down is not fit to enter the science of Homœopathy. He must be innocent of these things; he must put that aside and be willing to learn of all sources, providing the truth flows from these sources. In this frame of mind, and this frame of mind only, can the physician proceed to examine the Materia Medica.

We have already said that Hahnemann had no Materia Medica to start with. He could not go to books, and read, and meditate, and find remedies in the image of human sickness. He had no such remedies to study, and hence it was necessary to build up the Materia Medica. We can imagine that Hahnemann must have been almost in a state of despair, and inclined to say there is no knowledge upon the earth. He felt in his own mind that we should never know anything about the Materia Medica so long as we perceived its effects only in human sickness, but that a true and pure Materia Medica must be formed by observing the action of medicines upon the healthy human race. Hahnemann did not commence to feed these medicines to others; he took the Peruvian Bark himself, and felt its effects upon himself. He allowed it to manifest its symptoms, and when he had thus proved Peruvian Bark (which we call China) it might be then said that the first remedy known to man was discovered, and that the first drug effect was known and that China was born! Hahnemann searched the literature of the day to find out what other effects of China had been discovered accidentally, and accepted such as were in harmony with what he had discovered. We have already referred to the fact that Hahnemann was able, after proving China, to see that in its action it closely resembled the intermittent fevers that had existed through all time; that there was the most abundant relation of similitude between China and intermittent fever. Do we wonder, then, that Hahnemann said to himself, can it be possible that the law of cure is the law of similars? Can it be possible that similars are cured by drugs that produce symptoms like unto the sickness? Every drug he proved thereafter established the law more and more, made it appear more certain, and every drug that he proved added ono more remedy to the instrument that we call the Materia Medica, until it came to be what we now recognize as Hahnemann's Materia Medica Pura and the Materia Medica of the Chronic Diseases. This work was simply enormous and very thorough, but many additions have been made to it since the time of its publication, and these form the instruments we have to examine.

The best way to study a remedy is to make a proving of it. Suppose we were about to do that; suppose this class were entering upon a proving. Each member of the class would devote, say, a week, in examining carefully all the symptoms that he or she is the victim of, or believes himself or herself to be the victim of, at the present time, and for many months back. Each student then proceeds to write down carefully all these symptoms and places them by themselves. This group of symptoms is recognized as the diseased state of that individual.

A master-prover is decided upon, who will prepare for the proving a substance unknown to the class and to all the provers, known only to himself. He will begin with the first or earliest form of the drug, it may be the tincture, and potentize it to the 30th potency, putting a portion of that potency into a separate vial for each member of the class. The provers do not know what they are taking, and they are requested not to make known to each other their symptoms. When their own original symptoms appear in the proving the effect of the remedy upon any one of these chronic symptoms is simply noted, whether cured or exaggerated, or whether or not interfered with; but when the symptom occurs in its own natural way, without being increased or diminished, it may be looked upon as one of the natural things of that particular prover, and hence all the natural things of the prover are eliminated. Generally if a remedy takes a marked hold of a prover all the chronic symptoms will subside, but when a proving only takes a partial hold it may only create a few symptoms. These few symptoms, when added to the symptoms that the other provers have felt, will go to make up the chronic effect of the remedy, which may be said to be the effect of the remedy upon the human race. Now as to the method.

After the master prover deals out these vials, each prover takes a single dose of the medicine and waits to see if the single dose takes effect. If he is sensitive to that medicine a single dose will produce symptoms, and then those symptoms must not be interfered with; they should be allowed to go their own way. In the proving of an acute remedy, like Aconite; the instructor, who knows something about the effect of the medicine, may be able to say to the class: "If you are going to get effects from this remedy you will get those effects in the next three to four days." It will not be necessary to wait longer than that for Aconite, Nux Vomica, or Ignatia, but longer for Sulphur or some of the antipsorics. If we were attempting to prove a remedy like Silicate of Alumina, the master-prover would advise the class not to interfere with the medicine for at least thirty days, because its prodrome may be thirty days.

It is highly important to wait until the possible prodrome of a given remedy is surely passed. If it is a short-acting remedy, the action will come speedily. We must bear in mind the prodrome, the period of progress and the period of decline when studying the Materia Medica as well as when studying miasms. The master-prover will usually be able to indicate to the class whether they should wait a short time or a long time before taking another dose, and from this the class will only know whether the drug to be proved is acute or chronic.

If the first dose of medicine produces no effect, and enough time has been allowed to be sure that the prover is not sensitive to it, the next best thing to do is to create a sensitiveness to it. If we examine into the effects of poisons, we find those who have once been poisoned by Rhus are a dozen times more sensitive than before. Those who have been poisoned by Arsenic are extremely sensitive to Arsenic after they allow the first effects to pass off. If they continue, however, to keep on with the first effects they become less sensitive to it, so that they require larger and larger doses to take effect. This is a rule with all poisonous substances that are capable of affecting the human system markedly. Now, when the time has passed by which the prover knows he is not sensitive to that remedy, that he has not received an action from the dose (and perhaps in the class of forty you will not get more than one or two that will make a proving from the 30th potency) to make the proving and to intensify the effect, dissolve the medicine in water and have him take every two hours for 24 to 48 hours, unless symptoms arise sooner. By this means the prodromal period is shortened. The medicine seems to be intensified by the repetition, and the patient is brought under the influence, dynamically, of that remedy. As soon as the symptoms begin to show, it is time to cease taking the remedy.

No danger comes from giving the remedy in this way; danger comes from taking it for a few days and then stopping it, and then taking it again. For instance, say you are proving Arsenicum; you find that you are not all sensitive to it, and after waiting thirty days you start out again and take it in water, for three to four days, and the symptoms arise : now wait. So long as you discontinue it, it will not do any damage. Now, the symptoms begin to arise; wait, and let the image-producing effect of Arsenicum wear off; let it come and spread and go away of itself; do not interfere with it; if you do interefere with it, the interference should be only by a true antidote; you should never interfere with it by a repetition of dose. That is one of the most dangerous things. If the Arsenic symptoms are coming and showing clearly, and at the end of a week or ten days you say: "Let us brighten this up a little, and do this thing more thoroughly," and to accomplish this you take a great deal more, you will engraft upon your constitution in that way the Arsenicum diathesis, from which you will never be cured. You are breaking right into the cycles of that remedy and it is a dangerous thing to do. At times that has been done and the provers have carried the effects of their proving to the end of their days. If you leave this Arsenical state alone it will pass off entirely, and the prover is very often left much better for it. A proving properly conducted will improve the health of anybody; it will help to turn things into order. It was Hahnemann's advice to young men to make provings.

Another portion of the class will not get symptoms, no matter how they abuse the remedy, and if it be Arsenicum they will have to take a crude dose of it to get any effect, and then the symptoms given forth are only the toxic effects, from which little can be gained. The toxicological results of poisons are provings of the grossest character: they do not give the finer details. For instance, you give Opium in such large doses that it immediately poisons; you see nothing but the grosser, overwhelming symptoms; the irregular, stertorous breathing, the unconsciousness, the contracted pupil and the mottled face and the irregular heart. The details are not there, you only have a view of the most common things.

The reproving of remedies is of great value. The Vienna Society did not fully endorse Hahnemann's provings. This society thought it impossible that such wonderful things could be brought out upon the sensations of people. The society did not endorse the 30th potency that was recommended by Hahnemann for proving. So this society gathered itself together and resolved to prove remedies, and to test the 30th potency, and it so happened that the society was honest. Natrum mur., Thuja and other remedies were proved, and W—was honest enough to say that although his convictions were decidedly against the provings he had to admit that the symptoms gathered from the 30th potency were very strong. The Vienna Society demonstrated by these reprovings that the polychrests of Hahnemann had been fully proved. Their provings of the 30th of Natrum mur. was a wonderful revelation of them; but W—, in spite of this result, held on to his prejudices. He acknowledged that he was wrong; but he continued to use potencies lower than the 15th. He could not get his mind elevated to the 30th; his prejudice was too strong. Dunham says of some of these, that in spite of the fact that they had seen better results from the 30th and higher potencies even, they were so prejudiced they could not bring themselves to a state of yielding. As Dunham humorously expressed it, "they are ossified in their cerebral convolutions as well as in their bony structure." That is to say, their minds were inelastic, they could not expand. We talk from appearance when we say the eyes are closed; it is the mind that is closed, the understanding that is closed.

Read § 107-112.—When the patient is under the poisonous influence of a drug it does not seem to flow in the direction of his life action, but when reaction comes then the lingering effects of the drug seems to flow, as it were, in the stream of the vital action. Then the symptoms that arise are of the best order, and hence it is necessary in proving a drug to take such a portion of the drug only as will disturb and not suspend, as it will flow in the stream of the vital order, in the order of the economy, establishing slightly perverted action, and causing symptoms, without suspending action, as we would, for example, with a large dose of Opium. When a state of suspension exists in the dynamic economy, then we have a beclouding of all the activities of the economy; so giving a large dose of medicine to palliate pains and sufferings is dangerous. We have a suspension of the vital order when we give a medicine that does not flow in the stream of the vital influx, Homœopathy looks towards the administration of medicines that are given for the purpose of either creating order, and then always in the higher potencies, or for the purpose of disturbing, and then in the lower potencies. We should never resort to crude drugs for provings, unless for a momentary or temporary experiment. It should not be followed up, and no great weight should be put upon the provings that are made from the crude medicines. They only at best give a fragmentary idea. Unless the proving that has been made with strong doses becomes enlarged with the symptoms from small doses the information remains fragmentary and useless. If we had only the poisonous effects of Opium, we would be able only to use it in those conditions that simulate the poisonous effects of Opium, like apoplexy.

There are some prescribers who teach that for the primary effect one potency must be used and for the secondary effect another must be used. No such distinction need be made. I have many times been at the bedside of apoplectic patients when death would have followed had not the homœopathic remedy been administered. I have been at the bedside of some when the pulse was flickering, when the eye was glazed, when the countenance was besotted, stertorous breathing coming on, frothing at the mouth, and in a few minutes after the administration of Opium c.m. I have seen the patient go into a sound sleep, remain quiet and rest, wake up to consciousness, and go on to recovery. Alumina has a similar state of stupor resembling apoplexy, and hence it is that Alumina and Opium are antidotes to each other. I remember a case of apoplexy once that puzzled many physicians for some days, and I was puzzled, too. The patient was in a profound stupor. Opium was administered by the physician in charge before I arrived, and it stopped the stertorous breathing, but the patient remained unconscious. Finally it was observed that one side was moving, whilst the other side had not moved for many days, and that on the paralyzed side there was fever, while on the well side there was no fever. That was observed after careful examination for many days. I asked the doctor if he did not consider that the natural state of a paralyzed side would be coldness; he thought so too. The whole paralyzed side of this patient had a feverish feeling to the hand, the other side was normal. That seemed to be the only strange thing in the case; no speech, no effort to do anything, no action of the bowels; a do nothing case. Upon a careful study of the Materia Medica, I came to the conclusion that Alumina was suited to the case, and in twelve hours after taking a dose of Alumina in a high potency that fever subsided on the paralyzed side and the patient returned to consciousness.

LECTURE XXIX

IDIOSYNCRASIES

§ 17. The study of the *idiosyncrasies* is closely related to Homœopathy. The usual explanation of the term is, an oversensitiveness to one thing or a few things. It does not apply to the general susceptibility in feeble constitutions where patients are susceptible to all things, over-susceptible and over-impressed by simple annoyances. In the old school idiosyncrasies relate to certain patients who are known in every practitioner's practice as oversensitive. One oversensitive cannot take Opium for his pains, because of the congestion it produces, because of dangerous symptoms; he is oversensitive to it and has complication from a very small dose even and the physician is compelled not to administer it. Another patient connot tolerate Quinine in chills and fever; the primary action of Quinine makes him alarmingly sick; where another individual may take 15 grains. One who has an idiosyncrasy to Quinine cannot take one-quarter of a grain without having an over-action of that drug —a state of quininism. The homœopath recognizes of wide range in susceptibility, including things that the allopath is not acquainted with. There may be a chronic idiosyncrasy from a chronic miasm and an acute idiosyncrasy from an acute miasm. There are certain individuals in every community that cannot ride in the country because of their susceptibility to hay fever; others cannot bear the smell of flowers in the room because of becoming sick; some will get sick from the smell of roses. I have known a number of patients who became sick in this way. It is common enough, and the sickness is known by the name of rose cold or rose fever. I have a patient who cannot have dry lavender flowers in the house without coming down with coryza. She is disturbed by two or three things in this way, and will go looking about to see which one of those things is in the house. I had another patient who could not have peaches in the room without becoming sick; one of the symptoms that he had was diarrhœa. This oversensibility is very important and it explains in a measure the susceptibility to the remedy that will cure. If an idiosyncrasy to the remedy is not present, the patient will not be susceptible enough to be cured. The state in which he becomes sensitive enough to a drug to cure him is very analogous to these idiosyncrasies above mentioned. Think what susceptibility man must have to the remedy that cures him, when it cures in the very high attenuations that we use.

There are acquired idiosyncrasies and idiosyncrasies that are born with a patient. Those that are congenital and those that come from poisons are most difficult. In Rhus tox. poisoning those that have once been affected by handling it are so sensitive to it that if they go within a quarter of a mile of the vine, though they cannot detect it with the nose, yet in a few days they will come down with a case of Rhus poisoning. A very high potency of Rhus will sometimes remove that susceptibility and a dose of Rhus c.m. or m.m. will often check the acute poisoning from Rhus: but if you find that the patient has been born with a sensitivity to Rhus, while Rhus may palliate a few times it will finally cease to help him. When one is born with this sensitivity it is very tenacious and will sometimes persist, in spite of our best endeavors, to the end of life. If eradicated at all, it requires an antipsoric to get to the bottom of it. Hay fever is brought on in the fall and is supposed to be caused by the patient's over-sensitiveness to irritants that develop about that time; sometimes it is attributed to the hay that is curing in the fields at that time, sometimes to the different weeds that grow up then. Such patients have often been able to ferret out the thing that they are susceptible to. But psora is at the bottom of all these troubles. Patients getting up from typhoid fever have often idiosyncrasies, and the chronic miasms are responsible for these, just as psora is prior to the sore eyes from scarlet fever. Sequelæ are miasmatic, they are simply the outcroppings of chronic miasms.

There are persons who are sensitive, not merely to one or a few things, but to all things; oversensitive to the high potencies, oversensitive in taste, oversensitive to light, and a great many other things. This is a constitutional state; the patient is born with it. There are persons in whom you will see the sensitiveness only when you go away from the plane of nutrition into the plane of dynamics. You will see for instance patients who will sit at the table and crave common salt; want lots of salt upon their food, and never seem able to get just exactly what they need. They eat plenty of common salt and remain sick, growing thinner all the time. This is on the nutritive plane; the crude common salt is taken with the food. Now you administer the c.m. to such a patient, and it makes that patient sick, producing a violent aggravation.

This is where a food sustains a curative relation upon a higher plane. We step out of the nutritive plane into the plane of dynamics, the plane of disease-cause and cure.

Take Calcarea as an instance. We see the allopath and crude medicine man give to certain babies, that are slow in forming bone and teeth and have open fontanelles, lime water in milk, and the more lime water he gives them the less bone they make. Here is a bone-salt inanition, a non-assimilation of lime. A dose of Calcarea very high will enable that child to take all the lime that it needs from the food that it eats. The remedy given on the dynamic plane cause a digestion and assimilation of the lime naturally present in the food. You may feed lime in crude form, and no benefit ever come; the child goes on withering and emaciating.

In such non-assimilating patients the symptoms of Calcarea or Natrum mur. appear, calling the attention of the intelligent physician to the fact that the child needs Calcarea or Natrum mur. We know very well that we do not build bone with the c.m. potency of lime, it simply corrects internal disorder and causes the outward forms of the body to flow into order. The turning into order of the internal establishes the nutritive principle from the internal to the external. So that we can see the wider ranges that idiosyncrasy or susceptibility has in Homœopathy.

Here we might undertake to coin a word, viz. : —homœopathicity; what does it mean? Homœopathicity is the relation between the homœopathic remedy and the patient who has been cured. When the homœopathic remedy has acted properly, when it has cured the patient, it has demonstrated that it was homœopathically related to the case; so that the relation, when it was sustained, may be called the homœopathicity, and it is demonstrated by administering the remedy. It is true that we can have what would be called a normal homœopathicity, a normal state, and that state exaggerated. That state exaggerated is where the patient is oversensitive to the curative remedy, and it not only establishes a curative relation, but before curing produces an exaggeration of the symptoms of the patient. A remedy demonstrates its similitude to a case by curing. Homœopathic physicians use the word simillimum. The simillimum might be called that remedy that has cured the patient, but in advance of curing that case it is only what *appears* to be the most similar; a medicine cannot be called the simillimum until it has cured.

It is worthy of consideration to discover the difference between a poison taken upon the nutritive plane, that is, in crude substance, and a poison taken upon the dynamic plane. A poison upon the nutritive plane is usually not very deep, is more superficial, it relates more to external things, to the body and tissues, while the poison taken upon the dynamic plane may last a lifetime. The miasms are of such a character. Poison taken upon the nutritive plane may bring about a life-long effect upon an individual, owing to susceptibility. The small doses of Arsenicum will establish an Arsenicum poisoning that will last a lifetime, but this is nowhere so deep as will be represented by the higher potencies of Arsenicum. To poison a patient with the higher potencies there is generally required something of susceptibility, while to poison patients upon the nutritive plane susceptibility is not required; any patient can be brought under the influence of a poison given upon the nutritive plane.

Here is another difference. Substances that are inert and substances that we can use as food on the nutritive plane may become poisonous upon the dynamic plane to those that are susceptible. So that there is no substance that may not be a poison in the higher and highest potencies. This gives us a distinction between crude and dynamic poisons that you will do well to think about.

Now from all this we are led to see that if there were no state of susceptibility, no such condition as idiosyncrasy, there could be no Homœopathy. If there were no susceptibility, there would be no sickness and no need of Homœopathy.

Susceptibility underlies all contagion and all cure. So that cause and cure, the cause of sickness and the cure of sickness, knock at the same door. They flow in the same way because of the immaterial or simple substance. All disease is in primitive substance, or first substance; all cure of disease must also be in simple substance. In olden times we used to think that all substances capable of extinguishing the vital force, or which overcome the vital force, were poisons; that in itself is a crude idea of a poison. Any substance capable of impressing itself upon the economy of man sufficiently to cause death, or to create a disorder in the economy, may be called a poison. The difinition will apply to both dynamic and crude poisons. Poison presents two problems: an external problem and an internal problem. The external deals with the question of quantity, the internal with the question of quality. A dynamis cannot be considered from the standpoint of weights and measures, but from quality. Crude substances are considered from the standpoint of quantity, from weights and measures.

This is only a beginning to set you thinking. This subject leads into the study of protection as well. There are two forms of protection from sickness. Man is protected from sickness in two ways, by Homœopathy and by use. The physician and the nurse who go into the district of yellow fever or typhoid or diptheria smallpox, who keep busy, who have, in the highest sense of the word, the true love of the use, who have gone into the work as mediums of mercy, will be largely protected just simply from their love of the work, from their delight in it. They have no fear. Fear is an overwhelming cause of sickness; those who fall prey to fear are likely to become sick, but those who face disease with no fear are likely to remain well; they do sometimes fall sick, it is true, but I believe it is because they begin to have fear in the work.

The other and greater prophylactic is the homœopathic remedy. After working in an epidemic for a few weeks, you will find perhaps that half-a-dozen remedies are daily indicated and one of these in a large number of cases than any other. This one remedy seems to be the best suited to the general nature of the sickness. Now you will find that for prophylaxis there is required a less degree of similitude than is necessary for curing. A remedy will not have to be so similar to prevent disease as to cure it, and these remedies in daily use will enable you to prevent a large number of people from becoming sick. We must look to Homœopathy for our protection as well as for our cure.

LECTURE XXX

INDIVIDUALIZATION

§ 118, etc. Comparison, individualization, and difference in the nature of things most similar, are points that must be carefully considered. The substitution of one remedy for another cannot be thought of, or entertained in Homœopathy. The homœopathic physician must individualize, he must discriminate. He must individualize things widely dissimilar in one way, yet similar in other ways. Take for instance the two remedies, Secale and Arsenicum; they are both chilly, but the patient wants all the covers off and wants the cold air in Secale, and he wants all things hot in Arsenicum. The two remedies thus separate at once; they are wholly dissimilar as to the general state, whilst wholly similar as to particulars. A mere book-worm symptom hunter would see no difference between Secale and Arsenicum. You go to the bedside of a case of peritonitis, and you will find the abdomen distended, the patient restless; you will find him often vomiting blood and passing blood from the anus; you will find horrible burning with the distended abdomen, unquenchable thirst, dry, red tongue, lightning-like pulse. Well, Arsenicum and Secale have all these things equally; they both have these things in high degree; but when Secale is indicated he wants all the covers off, wants to be cold, wants cold applications, wants the windows open; cannot tolerate the heat, and the warm room makes him worse. If Arsenicum is indicated in such a case, he wants to be wrapped up warmly, even in the month of July, wants hot food and hot drinks. The whole Materia Medica is full of these things and is based upon this kind of individualization.

Without the generals of a case no man can practice Homœopathy, for without these no man can individualize and see distinctions. After gathering all the particulars, one strong general rules out one remedy and rules in another. Physicians by the questions they ask often show that they have not been able to grasp this idea of individualization. They pick out two symptoms, or one symptom common to two remedies, and say, "Now, both of these remedies have this same symptom, how are you going to tell them apart?" Well, if you are acquainted with the Materia Medica, with the art of individualization, you will at once easily see how to get the generals; the generals of one are so and so, and the generals of the other are so and so, and this will enable you to distinguish one of these remedies as best adapted to the constitution, when the two remedies have the one symptom in any equal degree. Now, this rules out the idea of substitution. If one does not work, they say, try all down the list alphabetically, until you hit it. Why a remedy that has never been known to produce that symptom may cure the case, because it is more similar to the *generals* of that case than any other. This is the art of applying the Materia Medica. Many times a patient brings out that which is so strange and rare that it has never been found in any remedy. You have to examine the whole case and see which remedy of all remedies is most similar to the patient himself. From beginning to end, the homœopath must study the patient. If he become conversant with symptoms apart from the patient, he will not be successful.

Par. 118 reads: "Each medicine produces particular effects in the body of man, and no other medicinal substance can create any that are precisely similar." That is the beginning of a doctrine showing that there can be no substitution. There are cases that are so mixed that man, no matter how much he studies, cannot see the distinctions; but, remember one thing, there is one remedy that is needed in the case, whether it is known or not; it is needed in the case, and it has no substitute, for that remedy differs from all other medicines, just as this individual differs from all other individuals. It may be that we cannot see that it is needed, it may not appear to be indicated, but it is needed all the same, though the intimation may not have come to the eye or ear of the physician. That shows the necessity of waiting and watching. In Homœopathy medicines can never replace each other, nor one be as good as another.

As we hasten along with this subject, we find in Par. 122 Hahnemann says: "In circumstances of this nature on which depend the certitude of the medical art, and the welfare of future generations, it is necessary to employ only medicines that are well-known." Purity is important, medicines as they are proved should be kept unmodified and preserved and possessed of their full energy. Now, it is important that you shall use the same substances, as nearly as possible, as were proved. Among the potencies that we are using here as high potencies, made by Fincke and others, we have in a large number of instances the very identical substances that were proved by the provers. It is important not to change. A plant bearing the same name as the one proved, but grown in a different climate and on a different soil, should not be used. Procure the one that was proved originally. Fincke recognized this when he procured the substances that Hering proved. We have the same Lachesis that Hering proved. I have a sample of the original Lachesis that I am preserving in a little vial marked with Hering's own name. The medicine should be well-known; its history should be well-known, with all the steps and details. The question of potentization should be taken into account, the different hands they have been through; all the little particulars of our high potencies should be well known. You should not be careless in this and not gather potencies from Tom, Dick and Harry. When able, go to headquarters and get your potencies.

Hahnemann writes in Par. 144: "A Materia Medica of this nature shall be free from all conjecture, fiction or gratuitous assertion—it shall contain nothing but the pure language of nature, the results of a careful and faithful research." We have formed, built and established the Materia Medica by provings upon the healthy, and observations that are pure and honestly made. Par. 145: "We ought certainly to be acquainted with the pure action of a vast number of medicines upon the healthy body, to be able to find homœopathic remedies against each of the innumerable forms of disease that besiege mankind; that is to say, to find out artificial morbific powers that resemble them." At the present time it will rarely be found that a fully developed disease has not its simillimum, its remedy and cure, in our Materia Medica. It is only those mixed cases that are not developed that puzzle us.

LECTURE XXXI

CHARACTERISTICS

§ 146: "The third point in the duty of the physician is to employ those medicines whose pure effects have been proved upon a healthy person in the manner best suited to the cure of natural diseases homœopathically." We will take this up in our next talk. This third point in the duty of the physician referred to in Par. 146 really takes up the balance of the *Organon*.

Par. 147: "Of all these medicines that one whose symptoms bear the greatest resemblance to the totality of those which characterize any particular natural disease ought to be the most appropriate and certain homœopathic remedy that can be employed; it is the specific remedy in this case of disease." It is not an uncommon thing in this advanced day of science to read of specific remedies. The old school distinctly affirms that there are only three or four species, but almost every off-shoot who starts at something for himself has to a great extent the idea of specifics in him. One of the first things the quack physician seems inclined to do is to commence advertising specifics for headache, for diarrhœa, for this or that. This is altogether opposed to Homœopathy. There are no specifics in Homœopathy except at the bedside of a patient when the remedy has been wrought out with great endeavor and care. Then it may be said that that medicine which is found to be similar to the symptoms which characterize this disease is specific.

Now, please note that there is an emphatic sense in that word "characterizes." It is no ordinary expression. We have read in the earlier portions of the *Organon* that the disease makes itself known to the physician by signs and symptoms, and that the totality of the symptoms is the sole representation of the disease, to the physician; but that totality has to be studied to ascertain what there is, among all the symptoms, that *characterizes* the disease, or marks the symptoms as peculiar.

Now Hahnemann commences to analyze the totality of the symptoms for the purpose of giving it character. It has been said in these lectures that it is necessary to do that, that the information that leads up to characterizing is really the information that makes the homœopathic physician wise, by which he has the ability to intelligently understand that which he has to treat. That medicine which is best adapted is the most similar, but you cannot demonstrate beforehand that it is the specific homœopathic remedy; for you may be deceived in your idea of the nature of the case. But when that remedy has acted, then it may be seen that that remedy was homœopathic, or specific, or that it was not homœopathic. You have no idea as to what remedy will be homœopathic to the case until you have examined all the symptoms, and then proceed to find out that which characterizes.

Put that word *characterizes* in large type, in red letters. You cannot dwell sufficiently long upon that, because it grows greater and grander with every study of the case, that idea of the characteristic. What is there in this case which makes it an individual, what is there in it that makes it unlike any that ever existed? In the case of the remedy ascertain that which characterizes it. When these two occur before the perception, before man's mind, so that he can think upon them, and he realizes that the remedy is the most similar of all in the Materia Medica, then he is assured that that remedy will cure, and it only requires to be administered to prove that it is the specific. The homœopathicity is thus sustained, the similitude has been borne out by the medicine having cured. We cannot have the demonstration that the remedy is homœopathic until it cures the sick man; we may only presume that it is homœopathic, or say it appears to us that it is homœopathic, because that which is characteristic of the disease is most similar of all other things to that which is characteristic of that remedy, or vice versa. We may reasonably assume that that remedy is the specific, but the homœopathicity can ony be demonstrated by cure. So it does not make a remedy homœopathic simply to be carried in my case. Homœopathic remedies are not homœopathic simply because they have been used by a homœopath. Remedies are not homœopathic because potentized and attenuated or prepared after the fashion of our school.

What constitutes a remedy homœopathic? The answer is: It has demonstrated its curative relation to the patient, after having been prescribed in accordance with his symptoms, the recovery taking place in the proper direction, from above downward, from within out, and in the reverse order of the symptoms. That constitutes a remedy homœopathic, and that constitutes the prescription homœopathic. It is then a specific remedy, and in no other sense can a remedy be called a specific. Hahnemann gives his theory of cure in paragraph 148, but you are not compelled to adopt it. Hahnemann himself says it is only a theory, and he offers it as simply the best in view, but not as binding upon you to accept.

But Par. 149 is something that must be accepted, that is, it must be known, and then accepted because it is true. It is a general statement of the results of the homœopathic remedy in the cure of disease. The rejection of this paragraph must effect a separation amongst those who do not believe, and those who do believe. "When a proper application of the homœopathic remedy has been made, the acute disease which is to be cured, however malignant and painful it may be, subsides in a few hours, if recent, and in a few days, if it is somewhat older," etc.

From this I am placed under the plain necessity of acknowledging that if under my treatment such diseases do not subside, I have not found the right remedy. That will force the honest homœopathic physician to seek the proper remedy. Let not the blame be placed upon the failure of the system and of law and order, but let it be placed upon the one who practises it. Just so sure as you find the homœopathic remedy in a case of scarlet fever, just so sure you will see that fever fall and that child improve; while the rash will remain out, nothing of the malignancy of the case will remain, in an ordinary case of scarlet fever; we find that in a few days the child is so much better he wants to go to school. But then we treat the child and not the fever. Just so sure as the physician has in mind the rash of scarlet fever or of measles as the main element of the disease, he will make a failure, and the patient will not recover so speedily; but as a matter of fact, the homœopathic physician prescribes for the patient on that which characterizes the sickness, even though it be what is called a self-limiting disease.

§ 150. This treats of one of the difficulties we have to contend with. "If a patient complains of slightly accessory symptoms which have just appeared, the physician ought not to take this state of things for a perfect malady that seriously demands medicinal aid," etc., etc. It is right for you, when your patients are under constitutional treatment, to prescribe for a cold, but only when it is not an ordinary one. If the cold is likely to cause serious trouble, then you must prescribe for it; slight indisposition, however, should not receive remedies. You will have patients that will come to you at every change of the wind, at every attack of snuffles the baby has, at every little headache or every little pain. If you then proceed to change your remedy or prescribe for each one of these little spells of indisposition, you will, in the course of a little while, have such a state of disorder in the individual that you will wonder what is the matter with this patient. You had better give her no medicine at all, and if she is wise and strong and can feel confidence you can say to her that she does not need medicine for this attack; but occasionally give her a dose of constitutional medicine when these little attacks are not on. While you are young and cannot hold these patients with an iron grasp, when they come to you, you had better give them placebo, and let the indisposition pass off of itself. Watch it, however, and it may at the close develop some constitutional manifestations and throw light upon the patient that you have been treating. On the other hand, it is an easy matter to prescribe for severe acute diseases; they are decisive, they strongly manifest their symptoms, they are sharp cut in their expressions, the symptoms are prominent, and you will not be confused as you will be in the slight indispositions. The slight indispositions are nondescript, you do not know what to do for them. In vain you seek to find that which characterizes them, and hence it is doubtful about any remedy that is administered being of any value. You will be astonished after prescribing a number of years, and your patients have gained confidence in you, that when they come in with these little trivial ailments they won't have them after a few powders of sugar. They will say: "Doctor, my trouble went off splendidly." This is what is meant by letting the little things alone. Severe diseases exhibit a strong degree of symptoms, and hence you have something to do. Par. 151. "But if the few symptoms of which the patient complains are very violent, the physician who attentively observes him will generally discover many others which are less developed and which furnish a perfect picture of the malady."

LECTURE XXXII

THE VALUE OF SYMPTOMS

Nature of Symptoms {
- General
- Common
- Particular

Grades of Symptoms {
- General {
  - First Grade
  - Second Grade
  - Third Grade
- Common {
  - First Grade
  - Second Grade
  - Third Grade
- Particular {
  - First Grade
  - Second Grade
  - Third Grade

§ 153 is the one that teaches more particularly how the process of individualization or discrimination shall be carried out. It treats of characteristics, it treats of grades. The homœopathic physician may think he has his case written out very well, but he does not know whether he has or not until he has mastered the idea of this paragraph. He may have page after page of symptoms, and not know what the remedy is, and if he takes the record to a master the master will say: "You have no case!" "Why, I have plenty of symptoms." "But you have no case. You have left your case out; you have left the image of the sickness out, because you have failed to get anything that characterizes it. You have plenty of symptoms, but have not anything characteristic. You have not taken your case properly." Now, after you have mastered this paragraph you will know whether you have taken your case properly, you will know whether you have something to present to a master, a likeness of something. The lack of this knowledge is the cause of non-success with the majority homœopathic physicians. There are a great many homœopathic physicians that prescribe and tinker a long time with their cases, and will ask you what a characteristic is, and if it is some one peculiar thing that guides to a remedy. The idea of a keynote comes to the mind of many.

I do not mean that all or any part of what you have written is useless, but it is necessary to have individualizing characteristics to enable you to classify that which you have, to perceive the value of symptoms, and, if you must settle down to a few remedies, to ascertain which of these is more important than another, or most important of all. You cannot individualize unless you have that which characterizes. The things that characterize are things to make you hesitate, to make you meditate. Suppose that you have been acquainted with a large number of cases of measles, for instance, but along comes one of which you say to yourself, "That is strange; I never saw such a thing as that before in a case of whooping cough. It is peculiar." You hesitate, you meditate, and at once recognize it as something individual, because it is strange and rare and peculiar. You say, I do not know what remedy has that symptom. Then you commence to search your repertory, or consult those of more experience, and you find in the repertory, or upon consultation, that such a medicine has that thing as a strong feature, as a high grade symptom, and it is as peculiar in the remedy as in your patient, though you have never seen it before. You may have seen a hundred cases of measles without seeing that very thing. That peculiar thing that you see in measles relates to the patient and not to the disease, and as the sole duty of the physician is to heal the sick that peculiar thing will open the whole case to the remedy. When you find that the remedy has that symptom, along with the other symptoms, you must attach some importance to it, and when there are two or three of these peculiar symptoms they form the *characteristic features*.

What would you think would constitute a *common* symptom? We shall at once see that the common symptoms are those that appear in all cases of measles, that you would expect to find in measles. It would be strange to have measles without any rash; that would be peculiar. We know that the absence of rash is a striking state of affairs and means trouble, and is peculiar. Either it is not measles, or the absence of the rash is a serious state. Suppose it is a fever. The patient has intense heat, an ordinary fever coming in the afternoon and running through the night, with hot hands and feet, high temperature, dry tongue, etc. What would you say concerning the presence or absence of thirst? You would say it is *common* if he has thirst, because almost anybody who has fever would want water. Nothing is so natural to put fire out with as water, and the absence of thirst in a fever is strange, is rare and uncommon, peculiar and striking. You would ask yourself at once, is it not strange that he does not have thirst with such a high temperature? You at once strike to the remedies that are thirstless. You would not think of hunting up a remedy that has thirst.

So the absence of the striking features of disease constitutes a peculiarity that relates to the patient. Well, then, that which is pathognomonic is common, because it is common in that disease, but an absence of the pathognomonic characterizes that particular disease in that patient, and therefore means the patient, and in proportion as you have that class of symptoms just in that proportion you have things that characterize the patient, and the specific remedy for the patient will be the simillimum. It is necessary to know sicknesses, not from pathology, not from physical diagnosis, no matter how important these branches are, but by symptoms, the language of nature.

A true homœopathic prescription cannot be made on pathology, on morbid anatomy; because provings have never been pushed in that direction. Pathology gives us the results of disease, and not the language of nature appealing to the intelligent physician. Symptomatolgy is the true subject to know. No man, who is only conversant with morbid anatomy and pathognomonic symptoms, can make homœopathic prescriptions. In addition to diagnostic ability he must have a peculiar knowledge; that is, he must be acquainted with the manner of expression of each and every disease. He must know just how each disease expresses itself in language and appearance and sensations. He must know just how every remedy affects mankind in the memory and understanding and will, because there are no other things that the remedy can act upon as to the mind, and he must know how the remedy affects functions, because there are no other ways in which the remedy affects the body of man. Now, if he knows how diseases express themselves in signs and symptoms, then he knows what constitutes an individual disease a little different from all others. It is the peculiar way that the same disease affects different patients that makes the symptoms strange, peculiar and rare. That which is pathognomonic in the remedy is that which you will study out most, because it is that which is related to the patient. Such is the state of mind that the homœopathic physicians must keep themselves in in order to begin this study, and when they have begun to think in this way they can then study the symptoms of the disease as to grade.

The symptoms of the remedies must be studied especially with respect to *order on grade*. To look upon them as all alike, because they appear to be all on the same level, is to be unable to make distinctions. One symptom with some physicians is as good as another. It is a fact that symptoms, to a great extent, are upon a sliding scale. What is peculiar in one remedy is not in any degree peculiar in another. While it may be peculiar in a chronic case to have thirst, it is not so in a fever. That which is true in many respects in a chronic state may be the very opposite in an acute case. The chronic miasms are the very opposite in their character and order to the acute miasms, and this is a fact that the homœopathic physician must know.

If you had a striking case of inflammation of the parotid gland, the patient says: "Do not press upon it, because it is very sore," how would you classify that, as common or strange? If you think but a moment, you will see that it would be a very strange thing for a highly inflamed gland not to be sore, and that soreness upon pressure is not something to be prescribed for, but something to be known, to be taken into the general view of the case, and the remedy indicated in the case would be suitable if it have inflammation and soreness of the gland; there is nothing striking in that: quite a group of remedies have produced hardness, soreness and tenderness of the gland; it may be one of those, or it may be one which has never produced these things, if it have the characterizing features of the patient.

In sicknesses the symptoms that cannot be explained are often very peculiar; the things that can be accounted for are not so often peculiar; peculiar things are less known to man. For instance, a patient can sit only with his feet up on the desk, or with his feet elevated; he is a great sufferer, and because of this suffering he is compelled to put his feet up. The symptoms hence will be put down, worse from letting the feet hang down. "Well, what do you mean by that? Why, if I let my feet hang down, I find I bring the nates down upon the chair, and there is a sore place there." Now that is quite a different thing. You may find if it is an old man that he has a large prostate gland, which is very painful at times and very sore, and when he lets the feet hang down the gland comes in contact with the chair. So we see that the real summing up of the case is that this enlarged and sore prostate gland is worse from pressure, and all you have learned from that symptom is that the gland is sensitive to touch, which is a common symptom. There are instances, however, where by letting the feet hang down the patient is ameliorated; for instance, you take a periostitis and the pain is relieved by letting the limbs hang. No one can tell why that limb is better when hanging over the bed. He lies across the bed with the foot hanging over the side, and why it is that he cannot lie upon his back nobody can figure out. Now that condition is found in *Conium*, and you will not be astonished after you know that *Conium* has that symptom to find all the symptoms of your patient, say *Conium*. All the rest of them perhaps, are common.

Now, when you think along this line of science, it will not take you long to get into the habit of estimating among the symptoms that appear in a record the things that are common, the things that you would expect, and the things that are strange.

Again, we see that there are certain symptoms in the remedies that are *general* and on the other hand the symptoms that are general must also be taken into account in order to examine any record. All the things that are predicated of the patient himself are things that are general; all the things that are predicated of any given organ are things in particular. So we see how there are things in general, and things common, and things particular; some times it may be a condition or state, sometimes it may be a symptom. We have said that what the patient predicates of himself will generally appear to you to be at once something in general. When the patient says, "I am thirsty," as a matter of fact, although he feels that thirst in the mouth, yet it is his whole economy that craves the water.

The things of which he says, "I feel," are apt to be generals. The patient says, "I have so much burning," and if you examine him, you find that his head burns, that the skin burns, that there is burning in the anus, burning in the urine, and whatever region is affected burns. You find the word burning is a general feature that modifies all his sickness. If it were only in one organ, it would be a particular, but these things that relate to the whole of the man are things in general.

Again, when the patient tells things of his affections, he gives us things that are most general. When he speaks of his desires and aversions, we have those things that relate so closely to the man himself that the changes in these things will be marked by changes in his very ultimates. When the man arrives at that state that he has an aversion to life, we see that that is a general symptom and that permeates his economy; that symptom qualifies all the symptoms and is the very centre of all his states and conditions. When he has a desire to commit suicide, which is the loss of the love of his life, we see that that is very innermost. Medicines affect man primarily by disturbing his affections, by disturbing his aversions and desires. The things that he loved to do are changed, and now he craves strange things. Or the remedy changes his ability to comprehend, and turns his life into a state of contention and disturbance; it disturbs his will and may bring upon him troublesome dreams, which are really mental states. Dreams are so closely allied to the mental state that he may well say, "I dreamed last night;" that is a general state. The things that lie closest to man and his life, and his vital force, are the things that are strictly general, and as they become less intimately related to man they become less and less general, until they become particular.

The menstrual period gives us a state which we may call general. The woman says, "I menstruate," so and so; she does not attribute it to her ovaries or to her uterus; her state is, as a rule, different when she is menstruating. So the things that are predicated of self, of the *ego*, the things described as "I do so and so," "Dr., I feel so and so," "I have so much thirst," "I am so chilly in every change of the weather," "I suffocate in a warm room," etc., these are all general. The things that are general are the first in importance. After these have been gathered, you may go on taking up each organ, and ascertaining what is true of each organ. Many times you will find that the modalities of each organ conform to the generals. Sometimes, however, there may be modalities of the organs, which are particular that are opposed to the general. Hence we find in remedies that appear to have in one subject one thing, and in another subject the very opposite of that thing. In one it will be a general, and in another it will be a particular.

LECTURE XXXIII

THE VALUE OF SYMPTOMS (*Continued*)

It is very important that you should understand what is meant by general, common and particular symptoms and so I will repeat somewhat. The generals are sometimes made up of particulars. If you examine any part alone, you are only examining the particulars. If you examine the liver symptoms alone, you are examining particulars. If you are examining the eye symptoms, or the symptoms of any other region considered apart from the whole man, you are examining particular symptoms. But after you have gathered the particulars of every region of the body, and you see there are certain symptoms running through the particulars, those symptoms that run through the particulars have become generals, as well as particulars.

Things that apply to all the organs may be predicated of the person himself. Things that modify all parts of the organism are those that relate to the general state. Anything that the individual predicates of himself is also general. There are things that an individual might say of himself that might relate to only one organ, but of course that becomes a particular; but most of the things that the man predicates of himself are general.

Consider for instance, the symptoms of sleep. You might at first think that they relate to the brain, but the brain does not sleep any more than the whole man. "I was wakeful last night;" he is predicating something of himself and hence it is a general. Or, he says, "I dreamed;" well it is true that the whole man really dreamed. You might say that the mind merely dreamed, but the mind is the man, and, therefore, we see how important sleep and dreams become in the anamnesis of a case. Scarcely more important is what the woman says of her menstruation; menstruation so closely relates to the whole woman that it becomes most important. The special senses also are so closely related to the whole man that the smells that are grateful and the smells that are disagreeable become general.

There are certain smells that relate more particularly to the nose itself, because the smell is in the nose and is due to some pathological condition of the nose, and thus becomes a mere particular. The smell of food is agreeable when the man is hungry, and that will relate to the whole man, but one who has a vicious catarrh of the nose, with much local disturbance, has many perversions of smell, which are particular, because they relate to the nose. A patient says: "I see" so and so, without seeing; that relates to the generals. It is to a great extent a seeing with the understanding. Now, when the eye itself becomes affected, the symptoms gathered are particulars because they relate to the anatomy of the eye. The more the symptoms relate to the anatomy of the parts, the more external they are: the more they relate to the tissues, the more likely they are to be particular. But the more they relate to internals that involve the whole man, the more they become general.

The things, therefore, that relate to the man are the ones to be singled out in the anamnesis and marked first. After gathering together all the symptoms of a patient you should single out for study first of all everything and anything that you can predicate of the man, everything of which you can say *he* feels so and so, *she* suffers so and so. Find out what remedies relate to these symptoms first. Sometimes when you have figured the anamnesis of the generals, you have settled by your anamnesis upon three remedies, or possibly upon one. In ninety-nine cases of a hundred you can leave out the particulars, for the particulars are usually contained within the generals. If there be but one remedy that has the numerous generals, and covers those generals absolutely and clearly and strongly, that will be the remedy that will cure the case. There may be a lot of little particulars that may appear to contra-indicate, but they cannot; for nothing in particulars can contra-indicate generals. One strong general can over-rule all the particulars you can gather up. "Aggravation from heat" will throw out Arsenicum from consideration in any case.

It may be advisable to dwell again for a little upon the *common* symptoms. Sometimes we find in woman the common symptom, prolapsus. It is a common thing for them to say, "Doctor, I have such a dragging down in my bowels, as if my insides were coming out." That is a common feature, and it is a common symptom. There is nothing about that alone that will enable you to find a remedy, but for these common symptoms we have a class of remedies. When you see a rubric containing a dozen, fifteen or twenty remedies, you may often know it is a common symptom. We would say that all women who have prolapsus have to a great extent a dragging down feeling, as if the uterus would come out. If we were to take this symptom and follow it up, we would see that it works in various directions; we would see that it runs into generals, and into particulars. How shall we decide when to give *Sepia*, when *Lil tig.*, when *Murex.*, when *Bell.*, when *Puls.*, when *Nux*, and when *Natrum mur.*? To enable you to pick out of that group of remedies the one that will cure you must study both the generals and the particulars of the patient and the generals always first. If it be a *Nux vomica* patient who has the prolapsus of the uterus, what will she say of herself that will make you see *Nux* in it? She would be chilly; full of coryza, with stuffing up of the nose in a warm room; she would be very irritable, snappish, want to kill somebody, want to throw her child into the fire, want to kill her husband. She would probably have constipation and every pain she had with it would make her want to go to stool; urging to stool, but only a little is passed and she wants to go frequently. You see at once that she has the generals of *Nux*, and whatever particulars she has are in harmony with those generals, and so you go from generals to particulars. The whole problem, like any other scientific problem, must be gone into and followed from generals to particulars. Suppose that *Sepia* is indicated for that woman. You have in it as well this common symptom. Now, what is there in this patient that no other patient has? The dragging down is just the same, but with it an awful all-gone sinking feeling in the stomach, and she gets relief only when sitting with the legs crossed. She has a constant feeling of a lump in the rectum that makes her want to go to stool, but she goes for days without any urging at all; she is sallow and sickly, talks of bilious symptoms and has a yellow saddle over the nose. She tells that she has an aversion to her children, and feels very sad that she does not love her husband as she ought to. She is unable to exercise the love she has to her children. Now you have that which she says of herself in general, and that which she tells of the stomach and rectum in particular, and yet peculiar. You can see now that the dragging down sensation is not general nor particular, but is common.

Many of the symptoms of regions are both common and particular, particular because they are of regions and common because they describe a state. Scarlet fever gives us an illustration of this. We would group all the striking symptoms indicative of scarlet fever, the rash, the appearance of the mucous membranes, the sore throat, the fever, the history, and the period of prodrome. The remedies for scarlet fever must have these symptoms in common with scarlet fever. The appearance of scarlet fever is among the common things of *Belladonna*. *Ailanthus* has in its common things the appearance of scarlet fever; *Apis* has the appearance of scarlet fever; *Rhus* has the appearance of rough scarlet fever. *Sulphur* and *Phosphorus* have a rash similar to scarlet fever. So if we were to make a rubric for the repertory we would put the names of all these remedies in the common group and call it scarlet fever.

But when are you going to give one remedy and when another? We can sometimes figure out from local manifestations things in general. For instance, you can take an *Arum triph* patient; that which appears to be most striking is that he picks his nose and lips until they bleed. If you examine that state well you will ascertain that these parts and the fingers and toes tingle; about the extremities where the circulation is feeble and where the nerves are abundant, in the nerves of the fingers and toes, there is an unusual tingling like the creeping of ants, and he keeps picking at these parts. It is a state marking almost the whole economy. If you watch a little more closely, you will see that liquid oozes out of the parts he has picked, a bloody, watery oozing, and that it denudes the skin around the parts. It becomes a part of the general state. Then in scarlet fever, with the rash only partly out, we want to take the language of nature alone. I spoke of *Phosphorus*. *Phos.* has a typical scarlet fever rash. Suppose you have a case that is putrid, the rash has become very dusky and the skin has become mottled and purplish, and there are places about the body that have a tendency to suppurate. You find there are swellings about the neck, swellings upon the hands and fingers, that are inclined to suppurate; or there is an ozzing round about them and pus is welling forth, and the case is so putrid and offensive that as soon as you enter the room you detect the horrible stench. If you examine into the case, you will see that the child cannot get water enough and cannot get it cold enough. The countenance is sunken, and the eyes are puffed and swollen and red. Blotches are appearing of a specific character intermingled with the scarlet fever blotches. There you have a *Phos.* case, and *Phos.* will stop the trouble immediately. Now, what have you gathered together? You have gathered together an evidence of the general state. You see running all through that case putridity and a zymotic state. You may have many cases of malignant scarlet fever, and you will find that you can manage them with your remedies as you would an unruly horse with reins.

Now as to the grades. The value of symptoms is divided into three grades. General symptoms are divided into three grades, first, second and third, and common symptoms and particular symptoms are divided into the same three grades. You will see in Bœnninghausen a fourth grade, but as a matter of fact these remedies do not form a grade; they are only probationary remedies, requiring demonstration by reproving and clinical confirmation.

The general symptoms of the first grade are such as all or the majority of provers state of themselves as a class of provers. For instance, take that symptom of Apis, "suffocation in a warm room;" all the provers of Apis, or nearly all were affected to a great extent in that way. All the provers of Pulsatilla were worse in a warm room. There can be no doubt about such symptoms for all the provers felt that state so strongly. Kali-hyd., Pulsatilla, Iodine and Apis are among those that have that symptom in the first grade, worse in a warm room, suffocation in a warm room. Now when those symptoms which have existed as generals among the provers come into the experience of the practitioner, and are confirmed by curing those states extensively, wherever administered, for years, then these remedies are fully entitled to this grade. When only one prover has recorded a certain symptom, it is doubtful whether that is a symptom from the action of the remedy, but when several provers have recorded the same symptom it becomes confirmed. When that symptom has been removed or cured by the remedy in the hands of a physician, it can then be said to have been verified. So symptoms are (1) recorded, (2) confirmed by reprovings, and (3) verified upon the sick. When several provers have observed that Puls. is worse in a warm room, and this is confirmed by other provers, and then verified by cure upon the sick, it immediately places Pulsatilla in the first grade of that general state. Suppose that it were something that was in relation to the bladder; Puls. has a symptom of frequent urination; now, that is immediately classified as a particular symptom because it relates to a region. Now, if all of these provers had irritable bladder when they took Puls. that would be a confirmation of it, and if it cures for years experience verifies it and it is then placed as belonging to Pulsatilla under the particulars, and marked in the highest grade. So with the symptom of bearing down, which also comes under *Pulsatilla;* that would be classed as a common symptom, but of the first grade.

Suppose now that there are more symptoms that have only been brought out by a few of the provers; they do not run through the whole family of provers, but they have been confirmed and occasionally verified; then you see they are not entitled to so much consideration and as a matter of degree they belong to the *second* grade, because not so strong as the first grade, which produces these symptoms upon everybody or nearly everybody. Of course, what is true of the generals will be true of common and particular. Then as to the *third* grade. Now and then a prover brings out a symptom and it has not yet been confirmed by reproving, but it stands out pretty strong, and seems to be worthy of a third place, or it has been verified by having cured sick folks, or on the other hand it is admitted as a clinical symptom. Sometimes close and careful observers have noticed that certain symptoms, not in the proving, have generally yielded to a certain remedy, and others have confirmed this clinical experience; these symptoms are admitted to go into the third grade. A great many of Bœnninghausen's fourth grade symptoms really belong to the third grade, because Bœnninghausen was very cautious with the symptoms that had never been verified. His fourth grade remedies include such as he had gathered from his clinical experience, and he was doubtful about the propriety of placing them in the third grade, and also those symptoms that occurred in the provers but had not proper confirmation or were not verified. He laid them, as it were, upon a shelf for approbation, to be hereafter proved or accepted.

LECTURE XXXIV

THE HOMŒOPATHIC AGGRAVATION

§ 154 (Last clause). "A disease that is of no very long standing ordinarily yields without any great degree of suffering to the first dose of this remedy," which is to say that in acute disease we seldom see anything like striking aggravation unless the acute disease has drawn near death's door, or is very severe, unless it has lasted many days, and breaking down of blood and tissue is threatened, or has taken place. Then we will see sharp aggravations, great prostration, violent sweating, exhaustion, vomiting and purging following the action of the remedy. I have seen most severe reaction which seemed to be necessary to recovery. Such a state in acute disease where it has gone many days without a remedy and a great threatening is present will be to an acute disease what many years would be to a chronic disease of long standing. Long standing means as a matter of progress; if we say a disease of much progress, or of considerable ultimates, we understand it better. If the disease has ultimated itself in change of tissue, then you see striking aggravations, even aggravations that cannot be recovered from, such as we find in the advanced forms of tissue change, e.g., where the kidneys are destroyed or the liver destroyed, or in phthisis, where the lungs are destroyed.

A disease ought always to be well considered as to whether it is acute or chronic. Where there are no tissue changes, where no ultimates are present, then you may expect the remedy to cure the patient without any serious aggravation, or without any sharp suffering, for there is no necessity of reacting from a serious structural change. Where there is a deep-seated septic condition, where pyæmia must be the result, you will find sometimes vomiting and purging. As a reaction of the vital force of the economy when order is established, this order, which is attended by reaction, as it were, commences a process of house cleaning. It does it itself, the drug does not do it; if a crude substance is used it is the action of the drug, of course, but the action of the dynamic drug is to turn the economy into order. So it is with chronic disease. When the chronic disease has not ultimated itself in tissue changes, you may get no aggravation at all, unless, perhaps, it be a very light excerbation of the symptoms, and that slight excerbation of the symptoms is of a different character. It is the establishment of the remedy as a new disease upon the economy instead of the reaction which corresponds to a process of house cleaning. Elimination must take place, as we know, probably from the bowels, or stomach, by vomiting, by expectoration, or by the kidneys, in those cases where everything has been suppressed.

It may look like an aggravation when you have had for years a limb paralyzed from a neuritis. Suppose, after you administer a remedy that goes right to the spot, that is in the very highest sense homœopathic, or truly specific, that paralyzed limb commences to tingle and creep like the crawling interiorly of ants, tingling sometimes from which he cannot sleep for days and nights. This is due to the reaction of the nerves of the part. They are called into new life, into activity. I have seen this in paralysis. You take, for instance, a child who has lain in a stupor for a long time, from inaction of the brain, the tingling that comes in the scalp, in the fingers and toes is dreadful, the child turns and twists and screeches and cries, and it requires an iron hand on the part of the doctor to hold that mother from doing something to hush that cry, for just so sure as that is done that child will go back into death. That is a reaction, so that all over the benumbed parts, or where the blood begins to flow into parts where the circulation has been feeble, where the nerves take on sensation again, we have reaction, which is but the result of that turning into order. That part has been benumbed and dead, and when circulation takes place in the part in order to repair its tissue we have reaction, which is attended with distress. If the physician cannot look upon that and bear it, he will have trouble. If he thinks it is an indication for another remedy he will spoil his case.

We must discriminate between that which is reaction and that which calls for a remedy. These things are only seen in Homœopathy, never in any other practice. Sometimes the physician will be driven to his wit's end in dealing with these reactions. It is sometimes a dreadful thing to look upon, and the physician may be turned out of doors. Let him meet it as a man; let him be patient with it, because the ignorance of the mother or the friends can be no excuse for his violation of principle, even once.

A disease of very long standing sometimes fails to yield without this aggravation and disturbance and turmoil in the economy, and the deeper it is the more tissue change you have to contend with, and the more wonderful and distressing and painful is this reaction. When a patient comes back after every dose of medicine with violent reaction, with violent aggravation of the disease, with violent aggravation of the symptoms, you know then that there is some deep-seated trouble. There is a difference between the ultimates of disease and absolute weakness of the vital force. There is such a state as weakness of the economy, and there is such a state as activity of the economy, with much tissue change. In feeble patients you may expect feeble reactions, or none at all after your remedy, but in the feeble cases they are of such character that you have few symptoms, and you can very seldom find a remedy truly specific.

For example, say you get a patient that is destined to go into consumption, a merely suspicious case. You administer the right remedy and a violent reaction comes, a foreshadowing of what he will go through years from now if he is not cured by the remedy. A shocking condition will come upon him; he may be frightened and come back and tell you that that was an awful dose of medicine, poison, etc. That is the remedy disease, those are the symptoms of the remedy foreshadowing the future of that case, because if that remedy was not similar enough to him it could not do such things, and it is because of the similitude of his state; and he may only have those symptoms in shadow. But the remedy cannot give him symptoms that he has not. It cannot give him symptoms that are not related to him except in those cases that are called oversensitives. Oversensitives, you know, are such as are capable of proving everything that comes along. You must know whether the patient is oversensitive and proving the drug, or whether he has a vigorous constitution and is getting an aggravation. The remedy will be exaggerated in oversensitives and sometimes in those of weakly constitution, especially those with a very narrow receding chin, those who have sunken eyes, those who have senility marked in the eyes.

The next paragraph continues this one to a certain extent. Par. 155. "I say without any degree of suffering, because when a perfect homœopathic remedy acts upon the body, it is nothing more than symptoms analogous to those of the disease laboring to surmount and annihilate these latter by usurping their place." This is only speaking from experience. Whenever Hahnemann makes such a remark he does not place any great value upon it, because it is a matter of opinion.

You will find as a general thing in acute diseases, that if a slight aggravation of the symptoms comes in a few minutes, you will hardly ever think of giving another dose. The remedy is so similar and searches so thoroughly that it is hardly ever necessary to repeat it. Now there are circumstances when it is necessary to repeat, but this is so difficult to teach, and so difficult to lay down rules for, that the only safe plan is to begin cases without repetition, to give a single dose and wait, and watch its effects. I very commonly give in vigorous, typhoid fever patients medicine in water, because it is a continued fever; but I watch and wait, giving it several days, and the slighest sign of the action of the remedy causes me to stop it always. I never vary from that. In a fever where the patient is feeble, to gain an immediate reaction that should never be done.

In a remittent fever the reaction may come in a very few hours, and the one dose should be the rule, while in a typhoid the reaction will seldom come in a few hours. It is a matter of a few days, and hence the repetition is admissible. In typhoids that are somewhat delicate never do such a thing. The more vigor there is in a constitution the more the remedy can co-operate with that vigor to bring about a safe and quick action.

The more feeble the patient the more cautious you should be about using the smallest dose you can give. In many chronic disease it is possible to bring about a reaction in the first night, hence the danger of repeating the remedy. If the delirium subsides, or a moisture comes upon the skin, and he slumbers placidly, the medicine should never be given beyond such a state. There are times in diphtheria when the repetition of the remedy will kill, and there are times when repetition will save life. I hope some day to be able to discover the principles.

§ 158. "This trifling homœopathic aggravation of the malady during the first few hours, the happy omen which announces that the acute disease will soon be cured, and that it will, for the most part, yield to a first dose." That a natural disease can destroy another by exceeding it in power and intensity, but above all things by its similarity, is the whole truth and nothing but the truth. So that when this slight aggravation occurs you will seldom, if ever, have to give another dose in an acute disease. When this aggravation does not come, when there is not the slightest aggravation of the symptoms, and the patient appears to be gradually better after the remedy, then it is that the remedy shows that it has not acted upon the same depth; and that relief may cease in the case of an acute disease, and when that relief ceases the reaction has ceased and then another dose of medicine is correct practice.

Relief that begins without any aggravation of the symptoms, does not last so long in an acute disease as when an aggravation has taken place. A slight action of the remedy over and above the disease is a good sign. Again, you will find if your remedy was not perfectly similar you will not get an aggravation except in over-sensitive patients, and then it is a medicinal aggravation. When you find that you get no aggravation of the symptoms in a good vigorous constitution, none at all, very often your remedy has been only partially similar and it may require two or three of such partially similar remedies to finish the case. If you will observe the work of ordinary physicians, you will notice they give two or three remedies to get their patients through where a master gives but one.

§ 159. "The smaller the dose of the homœopathic remedy, the slighter the apparent aggravation of the disease, and it is proportionately of shorter duration." This was written at the time of Hahnemann's experience with what might be called small doses, ranging from the lower potencies to the 30th and seldom much higher. He had had ample experience with the 30th, and occasionally with the 60th, but not with tremendous turmoil that comes from the very highest attenuations. It reads in the correct translation of it (this is incorrect here): "The smaller the dose is of the homœopathic medicine, the less and the shorter is the aggravation in the first hours." It might be considered to mean an apparent aggravation, or an apparent aggravation of the disease. Now Hahnemann observes, as you will find amongst several of his writings, that the disease itself is actually intensified and made worse by the remedy, if the remedy be precisely similar, but if we pass away from the crudity of the medicines, ranging up towards the 30th potency, we get a milder action, and it has a deeper curative action, and the smaller the dose of the homœopathic medicine the less and the shorter is the aggravation. The idea is that there is an aggravation in the first hours; that is a matter that the paragraph itself admits, and it is this aggravation that Hahnemannn is talking about.

It is sometimes true that after the third or fourth potencies of Belladonna in a violent congestion of the brain, the aggravation is violent, and if the medicine is not discontinued the child will die. The disease itself appears to be aggravated, the child seems to be so susceptible to Belladonna that it appears as it were to be added to the disease, but with the 30th potency, as Hahnemann observes, this aggravation is slight and of short duration. Now, in this we get an outside aggravation. It is the drug disease of the remedy added to the natural disease, an aggravated state of the disease caused by the drug. It is true sometimes, in spite of this aggravation, that the patient says somehow or other he feels better.

This aggravation is unnecessarily prolonged by giving too low potencies; it is also prolonged by a repetition of the dose. I recently observed a state that occurred from repetition. I sent a very robust young woman, twenty years old, a dose of Bryonia, to be taken dry on the tongue. However, she dissolved it in water, and was taking it at the end of the second day, when I was sent for, at which time she seemed to be going into pneumonia. She had a dry, harsh cough. "What is the matter with my daughter, doctor, is she going to die?" She was proving Bryonia. I stooped the Bryonia, and next morning she was well. This has been seen a great many times when the medicine was similar. If the medicine is not very similar, only partially similar it yet may be similar enough to cure, but you will not see the results that I am now speaking of; but when you make accurate prescriptions, and are doing your best work, you will see these things in the very best constitutions.

Of course, the explanation is that the patient is as sensitive to the medicine that will cure her as to the disease that she has. Diseased states, then, are made worse by unnecessary repetition and by the dose not being small enough, that is, by the dose being very crude. The third, fourth and sixth are dangerous potencies, if you are a good prescriber, If you are a poor prescriber, you will demonstrate but little of anything. You will naturally go to the higher and higher potencies for the purpose of departing from what seems to be a poisonous dose.

This action differs from the aggravation of a c.m. potency, during the latter the patient feels decidedly better. It is short, it is decisive, and only the characteristic symptoms of the disease are aggravated. The disease itself is not aggravated; the disease itself is not added to, and is not intensified, but the symptoms of the disease stand out sharply and the patient says, "I am getting better." The symptoms sometimes are a little alarming, but intermingled with this is a ray of light that convinces the patient from his innermost feelings that he is getting better. "I feel much better this morning," says the patient, though the symptoms may have been sharpened up.

§ 160. We are accused nowadays of having departed from IInhnemann. Hahnemann wrote of the 30th potency in one of the stages of his life, as sufficiently high and sufficiently low. We can easily see that it was in the earlier period of his investigations that he made the remark that potentizing must end somewhere. We are accused of departing from Hahnemann, because we give different doses from what Hahnemann gavo. Now I want to show you that this is not so. Read paragraph 279: "It has been fully proved by pure experiments that when a disease does not evidently depend upon the impaired state of an important organ *the dose of the homœopathic remedy can never be sufficiently small so as to be inferior to the power of the natural disease which it can, at least, partially extinguish and cure, provided it be capable of producing only a small increase of symptoms immediately after it is administered."* Now, if we go to the 200th potency and find that that will aggravate, if we go to the 50m. and find that that will aggravate, if we go to the cm., the mm., etc., and find that they will aggravate, that they still have the power to intensify the symptoms, the remedy has just the same curative power in it. If we have tho potency so high that it is not capable of producing an aggravation of the symptoms, we may then be sure that there is no medicinal power left. We are up to the 13mm. and the end is not yet.

Now we have never made the claim that every potency will suit everybody. The potency must correspond to the state of the patient. If we ever find a person who will be aggravated in his symptoms in the most positive and definite fashion, that potency will be verified. We have not departed from Hahnemann, but have acted in accordance with his doctrines. § 280. "This incontrovertible axiom, founded upon experience, will serve as a rule by which the doses of all homœopathic medicines, without exception, are to be attenuated to such a degree, that after being introduced into the body they shall merely produce an almost insensible aggravation of the disease. It is of little importance whether the attenuation goes so far as to appear almost impossible to ordinary physicians whose minds feed on no other ideas but what are gross and material. All these arguments and vain assertions will be of little avail when opposed to the doctrines of unerring experience."

Now, can there be any doubt of what Hahnemann meant when he speaks of the smallest dose? Can there be any doubt but that he means attenuation, and attenuation up and up until we reach that point in the attenuation that we do not observe a slight aggravation of the symptoms? In the note to paragraph 249, he says, "All experience teaches us that scarcely any homœopathic medicine can be prepared in too minute a dose to produce perceptible benefit in a disease to which it is adapted. Hence, it would be an improper and an injurious practice when the medicine produces no good effect or an inconsiderable aggravation of the symptoms, after the manner of the old school to repeat or increase the dose under the ideas that it cannot prove serviceable on account of its minuteness."

So the senses have no relation whatever to the minuteness of the dose. The medical man is inclined to measure doses from the standard of a poisonous dose. He will measure off a little less than that which would poison, and call that a dose. It must be seen, it must yet be visible. This is not the test that Hahnemann offers. He offers the test of the dose as one capable of producing a slight aggravation of the symptoms. We see he does not limit attenuation, but he practically teaches it is unlimited, and the end has never been found.

There is a generally prevailing idea all over, not among strict Hahnemannians, but among modern homœopaths in general, that the dose of medicine laid down by Hahnemann is too small to cure. It is a fatal error. An increase of the dose cannot make it more homœopathic. The similarity of the remedy is first, and the dose is second. But that the dose of medicine laid down by Hahnemann is too small to cure is a fatal error. We must see by the experience in the clinics, and by considering the wonderful things that we have gone over in the doctrines, that we have really very little to do with the dose, that there is a wonderful latitude in dosage, and that we cannot lay down any fixed rule as to the best potency to use.

It ought to be distinctly felt, from all we have gone over, that the 30th potency is low enough to begin business with in any acute or chronic disease, but where the limit is no mortal can see. We want to follow up the series, so that we may get the very internal states that exist in degrees in the medicine. The different potencies are distinct from each other, some are very far apart, yet invariably connected. It is a mistake for any homœopath to start out with the idea that the dose of medicine laid down by Hahnemann is too small to cure. It shows that his mind is of material mould, that it is inelastic and cannot yield to the higher observations, and not capable of observing and following higher and higher as true experience would lead. Unless man has truth in his mind his experiences are false. Truth in the mind is first and then experiences are good. If his mind is in a state of truth, experiences are true. You cannot trust the experiences of men who do not know what is true, neither can they be led into truth by these fallacious experiences.

LECTURE XXXV

PROGNOSIS AFTER OBSERVING THE ACTION OF THE REMEDY

After a prescription has been made the physician commences to make observations. The whole future of the patient may depend upon the conclusions that the physician arrives at from these observations, for his action depends very much upon his observations, and upon his action depends the good of the patient. If he is not conversant with the import of what he sees, he will undertake to do wrong things, he will make wrong prescriptions, he will change his medicines and do things to the detriment of the patient. There is absolutely but one way, and nothing can take the place of intelligence. If you talk with a great many physicians concerning the observations you have made after giving the remedy you will find that the majority of them have only whims or notions on this subject and see nothing after the prescription is made. These observations I am going to give you have grown out of much watchfulness, long waiting and watching. If the homœopathic physician is not an accurate observer, his observations will be indefinite; and if his observations are indefinite, his prescribing is indefinite.

It is taken for granted after a prescription has been made, and it is an accurate prescription, that it has acted. Now, if a medicine is acting it commences immediately to affect changes in the patient, and these changes are shown by signs and symptoms. The inner nature of the disease appears to the physician through the symptoms, and it is like watching the hands upon the clock. This watching and waiting and observing has to be done by the physician in order that he may judge by the changes what to do, and what not to do. It is true that the homœopath is not long in doubt in many instances what not to do. There is always an index that tells him what not to do. If he is a sharp and vigilant observer, he will see the index for every case. Of course, if a prescription is not related to the case, if it is a prescription that effects no changes, it does not take long to see what to do; much patient waiting for a foolish prescription is but loss of time, and that should be taken into account among the observations. The observations taken after a specific remedy has been given sufficiently related to the case to cause changes in the symptoms are those of value.

The changes are beginning, what are they like, what do they mean, to what do they amount? The physician must know when he listens to the reports of the patient what is going on. The remedy is known to act by the changing of the symptoms. The disappearance of symptoms, the increase of symptoms, the amelioration of symptoms, the order of the symptoms, are all changes from the remedy, and these changes are to be studied.

Among the commonest things that remedies do is to aggravate or ameliorate. The aggravation is of two kinds; we may have an aggravation which is an aggravation of the disease, in which the patient is growing worse, or we may have an aggravation of the symptoms, in which the patient is growing better. An aggravation of the disease means that the patient is growing weaker, the symptoms are growing stronger; but the homœopathic aggravation, which is the aggravation of the symptoms of the patient while the patient is growing better, is something that the physician observes after a true homœopathic prescription. The true homœopathic aggravation, I say, is when the symptoms are worse, but the patient says, "I feel better."

We must now go into the particulars concerning these states, as to the time and place, as to how the aggravation occurs, as to how the amelioration occurs, as to duration, etc. The aggravations and ameliorations, the directions of symptoms and many other things have to come up, and be observed and judgment has to be passed upon them.

First of all, the patient should be the aim of the physician, his whole idea should be centred upon the patient to determine whether he is improving or declining. We have to judge by the symptoms to know that this is taking place. Very often the patient will say, "I am growing weaker," and yet you may know that what he says is not true; so certainly can you rely upon the symptoms and their story, which is more faithful than the patient's opinion. Many times the patient will say, "Doctor, I am so much worse;" and yet you examine into his symptoms and you find that he is really doing very well. Just the moment that he finds out that you are encouraged, he feels better and rouses up and wants to eat.

By the symptoms, also, you can tell when the patient is really weaker, and if the symptoms are taking an inward rather than an outward course you will know, even if he is encouraged, that there is no encouragement for him. We have in the symptoms that which we can rely upon. In the old school we have nothing but the information of the patient. This is of little account after making a homœopathic prescription. The symptoms themselves must be corroborated. The patient's opinion must be corroborated by the symptoms. The symptoms do corroborate what the patients say in many instances, but the symptoms are the physician's most satisfactory evidence.

Another general remark needs to be made, namely, that we should know by the symptoms if the changes occurring are sufficiently interior. If the changes that are occurring are exterior, the physician must be acquainted with the meaning of them, so that he will know by that whether the disease is being healed from the innermost or whether the symptoms have merely changed according to their superficial nature. Incurable diseases will very often be palliated by mild medicines that act only superficially, act upon the sensorium, act upon the senses, and, though the hidden and deep-seated trouble goes on and progresses, and is sometimes made worse, yet the patient is made comfortable. So that by the symptoms we can know whether the changes that are occurring are of sufficient depth, so that the patient may recover. The direction that the symptoms are taking is sufficient to tell that, especially in chronic disease.

A patient walks into the clinic, somewhat stoop-shouldered, with a hacking cough that he has had for a good many years. You judge by his looks that he has been sick a good while; his face is sickly, he is lean and anxious, he is careworn, he is suffering from poverty and poor clothing and scanty food. Now, you examine all of his symptoms, and they clearly indicate that he needs an antipsoric, for the symptoms are covered by an antipsoric, and from the history of the case you know he has needed it a good while. Upon prolonged examination, the antipsoric you have in mind is strengthened. You now examine his chest, and discover he has not the expansion that he ought to have, and you detect the presence of tuberculosis, and by feeble pulse and many other corroborating symptoms you ascertain that the patient has been steadily declining.

You give the medicine and he comes back in a few days with quite a sharp aggravation of the symptoms; he has an increased cough, he has a night sweat, and he is more feeble. Now, the homœopathic physician likes to hear that; he likes to hear of an exacerbation of the symptoms; but this patient comes back in a week, and the aggravation is still present, and is somewhat on the increase, the patient is coughing worse, and the expectoration is more troublesome than ever, his night sweats have been going on; he comes back at the end of the second week and he is still worse, and all the symptoms have been worse since he took that medicine. He was comparatively comfortable before he took that medicine, but at the end of the fourth week he is steadily growing worse. There has been no amelioration following this aggravation, and he is evidently declining; he now cannot come to the office for he is so weak.

This, then, will be the *first observation—a prolonged aggravation and final decline of the patient*. What have we done? It has been a mistake, the antipsoric was too deep, it has established destruction. In this state the vital reaction was impossible, he was an incurable case. The question immediately comes up, what are you to do? Are you not going to give the homœopathic remedy in such cases? The patient steadily declines. If you are in doubt about such action of the remedies and making the patient worse, you will probably have an undertaker's certificate to sign before long.

In incurable and doubtful cases give no higher than the 30th or 200th potency, and observe whether the aggravation is going to be too deep or too prolonged. There are many signs in the chest in such cases to make a physician doubt whether he will give a deep remedy when organic disease is present. Of course this does not apply when things are only threatening, when you have fear of their coming, but when you are sure of their being present. In the instance given the probability is that the remedy has been too late, and it has attempted to arouse his economy, but turned to destruction his whole organism. Then begin, in such cases, with a moderately low potency, and the 30th is low enough for anybody or anything.

When the patient does not seem to be quite so bad as the one I have just described, you get him a little earlier in his history before the trouble has gone quite so far, and then if you administer this same very high potency in the same way you will make a second observation. Though the aggravation is long and severe, yet you have a final reaction, or amelioration. The aggravation lasts for many weeks, perhaps, and then his feeble economy seems to react, and there is a slow but sure improvement. It shows that the disease has not progressed quite so far; the changes have not become quite so marked. At the end of three months he is prepared for another dose of medicine, and you see a repetition of the same thing, and you may know then that that man was on the border land and had he gone further, cure would have been impossible. It is always well in doubtful cases to go to the lower potencies, and in this way go cautiously prepared to antidote the medicine if it takes the wrong course.

Then the *second observation* is, the *long aggravation, but final and slow improvement*. If, at the end of a few weeks, he is a little better and his symptoms are a little better than when he took the dose, there is some hope that finally the symptoms may have an outward manifestation whereby he will attain final recovery, but for many years you may go along with prolonged aggravations. You will find in such a patient there was the beginning of some very marked tissue change in some organ. We may know by observing the action of a remedy what state the tissues are in, as well as know something about the prognosis for the patient.

The *third observation* after administering the homœopathic remedy is, where the *aggravation is quick, short and strong with rapid improvement of the patient*. Whenever you find an aggravation comes quickly, is short, and has been more or less vigorous, then you will find improvement of the patient will be long. Improvement will be marked, the reaction of the economy is vigorous, and there is no tendency to any structural change in the vital organs. Any structural change that may be present will be found on the surface, in organs that are not vital; abscesses will form and often glands that can be done without will suppurate in regions that are not important to the life of the patient. Such organic changes are surface changes, and are not like the changes that take place in the liver, in the kidneys, in the heart and in the brain. Make a difference in your mind between organic changes that take place in the organs that are vital, that carry on the work of the economy, and organic changes that take place in structures of the body that are not essential to life. An aggravation quick, short and strong is one that is to be wished for and is followed by quick improvement. Such is the slight aggravation of the symptoms that occurs in the first hours after the remedy in an acute sickness, or during the first few days in a chronic case.

Under the *fourth observation*, you will notice a class of cases wherein you will find very satisfactory cures, where the administration of the remedy is followed by no *aggravation whatever*. There is no organic disease, and no tendency to organic disease. The chronic condition itself to which the remedy is suitable is not of great depth, belongs to the functions of nerves rather than to threatened changes in tissues. You must realize that there are changes in tissues so marked that the vital force is disturbed in flowing through the economy, and yet so slight that man with all of his instruments of precision cannot observe them. Under such circumstances we may have sharp sufferings, but cures may come about without any aggravation. We know then that if there is no aggravation the potency just exactly fitted the case, but here you have a course of things that you need not always expect. Though there is nothing but a true nervous change in the economy after a potency that is not suitable, either too crude, or too high, for that patient, you will have an aggravated state of the symptoms. In cures without any aggravation we know that the potency is suitable, and the remedy, the curative remedy, provided that the symptoms go off and the patient returns to health in an orderly way. It is the highest order of cure in acute affections, yet the physician sometimes will be more satisfied if in the beginning of his prescribing he notices a slight aggravation of the symptoms. The *fourth observation* then relates to cases in which we have no *aggravation, with recovery of patient*.

The amelioration comes first and the aggravation comes afterwards is the fifth observation. At times you will see sickly patients, fully as sick as the one I mentioned in the first or second instance, walk into your office and after long study you administer a remedy. The patient comes back in a few days telling you how much better he was immediately after taking the medicine, and now he has three or four days of what appears to be a decided improvement, a prompt action of the remedy. The patient says he is better, and the symptoms seem to be better; but wait, and at the end of a week or four or five days all the symptoms are worse than when he first came to you. It is not a very uncommon thing in severe cases, in cases of a good many symptoms, to have an amelioration of the remedy come at once; but whatever you may say, the condition is unfavorable.

Either the remedy was only a superficial remedy, and could only act as a palliative, or the patient was incurable and the remedy was somewhat suitable. One of these two conclusions must be arrived at, and this can only be done by a re-examination of the patient and by finding out whether the symptoms relate to that remedy. Sometimes you will discover that the remedy was an error; a further study of the case shows that the remedy was only similar to the most grievous symptoms, that it did not cover the whole case, that it did not affect the constitutional state of the patient, and then you will see that the patient is an incurable one and the selection was an unfavorable one. It is the best thing for the patient if the symptoms come back exactly as they were, but very often they come back changed, and then you must wait through grievous suffering for the picture; and the patient will wait better if the doctor confesses on the spot that the selection was not what it ought to be, and he hopes to do better next time. It is a strange thing how the patients will have an increase of confidence if the doctor will tell the truth. The acknowledgement of one's own ignorance begets confidence in an intelligent patient.

The higher and highest potencies will act in curable cases a long time. When I say act, I only speak from appearance; I should say they appear to act a long time, for the remedy acts at once and establishes a condition of order upon the patient, after which there is no use in giving medicine. This order will continue a considerable length of time, sometimes several months. The patient will get along just as well without any medicine, and get along better without that medicine that helped him than with it. In curable cases, whose prospects are good, they will go along for a long time, and become very much relieved of their symptoms. Now, if the patient comes back at the end of the first, second and third week and says he has done well, that he has been improving all the time from the cm. of *Sulphur*, but at the end of the fourth week he comes back and says, "I have been running down," the physician must then pass judgment. Has this patient done something to spoil the action of this medicine? Has he been on a drink? Has he handled chemicals? Has he been in the fumes of Ammonia? No, he has done none of these things.

This condition is really an unfavorable one. To have a medicine act but a few weeks, whereas it ought to act for months thereafter, will make you suspicious of that patient. If nothing has taken place to interfere with this medicine in his economy you may be suspicious of this case. This *sixth observation is too short relief of symptoms*. The relief after the constitutional remedy does not last long enough, does not last as long as it ought to. If you examine the third observation you find that there you have the quick aggravation followed by long amelioration; but in this, the sixth, you have the amelioration, but of too short duration. In instances where you have an aggravation immediately after, and then a quick rebound, you will never see, absolutely never see, too short an action of that remedy; or, in other words, too short an amelioration of the remedy. If there is a quick rebound, that amelioration should last; if it does not last, it is because of some condition that interferes with the action of the remedy; it may be unconscious on the part of the patient, or it may be intentional. A quick rebound means everything in the remedy, means that it is well chosen, that the vital economy is in a good state, and if everything goes well, recovery will take place.

In acute cases we may see this too short amelioration of the symptoms; for instance, a dose of medicine given in a most violent inflammation of the brain may remove all the symptoms for an hour, and the remedy have to be repeated, and at the end of that repetition we find only an amelioration of thirty minutes. You may make up your mind, then, that that patient is in a desperate condition, it is too short an amelioration. The action of *Belladonna* in some very acute red-faced conditions is instantaneous. In five minutes I have noticed the amelioration come, but the best kind of an amelioration is that which comes gradually at the end of an hour or two hours, as it is likely to remain. If it is too short an amelioration in acute cases, it is because such high grade inflammatory action is present that organs are threatened by the rapid processes going on. It is too short amelioration in chronic diseases, it means that there are structural changes and organs are destroyed or being destroyed or in a very precarious condition. These changes cannot always be diagnosed in life, but they are present, and an acute observer, who has been working earnestly for years, will often be able to diagnose the meaning of symptoms without any physical examination whatever, so that he can prophesy as to the patient. Such experiences of an intelligent physician in a family will cause them to look upon him as wiser than anyone else, for he knows all about their constitutions. This he acquires by studying their symptoms, the action of remedies upon them, and their symptoms after the medicines have been given. This enables him to know the reaction of a given patient, whether slow or quick, and how remedies affect each member of that family. This belongs to the physician, and he should be intelligent enough to know something about them when he has been treating them a little while. The old physician is in possession of this knowledge, while the student and the new physician have it all to learn.

Once in a while you will see *a full time amelioration of the symptoms, yet no special relief of the patient,* which is the *seventh observation.* There are certain patients that only gain about so much; there are latent conditions, or latent existing organic conditions, in such patients that prevent improvement beyond a certain stage. A patient with one kidney can only improve to a certain degree; patient with fibrinous structural change in certain places, tubercles that have become encysted and lungs capable of doing only limited work, will have symptoms, and these symptoms will be ameliorated from time to time with remedies, but the patient is only curable to a certain extent; he cannot go beyond and rise above such a state. Remember this after several medicines have been administered, and the amelioration of the case has existed often the full length of time of the remedies, but the patient has not risen above his own pitch in this length of time. The remedies act favorably, but the patient is not cured, and never can be cured. The patient is palliated in this instance, and it is a suitable palliation for homœopathic remedies.

Observation eight. Some patients prove every remedy they get; patients inclined to be hysterical, overwrought, oversensitive to all things. The patient is said to have an idiosyncrasy to everything, and these oversensitive patients are often incurable. You administer a dose of a high potency, and they will go on and prove that medicine, and while under the influence of that medicine they are not under the influence of anything else. It takes possession of them, and acts as a disease does; the remedy has its prodromal period, its period of progress and its period of decline. Such patients are provers, they will prove the highest potencies. When you find a patient that proves everything you give in the higher potencies go back to the 30th and 200th potencies. Such patients are most annoying. You will often cure their acute diseases by giving them the 30th and 200th, and you will relieve their chronic diseases by giving them the 30th, 200th and 500th potencies. Many of them are born with this sensitivity and they will die with it; they are not capable of rising above this over-irritable and over-wrought state. Such oversensitive patients are very useful to the homœopathic physician. After they get out of one proving they are quite ready to repeat it or go into another.

The ninth observation is the action of the medicines upon provers. Healthy provers are always benefited by provings, if they are properly conducted. It is well to observe carefully the constitutional states of an individual about to become a prover, and to write these down and subtract them from the proving. These symptoms will not very commonly appear during the proving; if they do, note the change in them.

The tenth observation relates to new symptoms appearing after the remedy. If a great number of new symptoms appear after the administration of a remedy, the prescription will generally prove an unfavorable one. Now and then the coming of a new symptom will simply be an old symptom coming up that the patient has not observed, and thinks it a new one. The greater the array of new symptoms coming out after the administration of a remedy, the more doubt there is thrown upon the prescription. The probability is, after these new symptoms have passed away, the patient will settle down to the original state and no improvement take place. It did not sustain a true homœopathic relation.

The eleventh observation is when old symptoms are observed to reappear. In proportion as old symptoms that have long been away return just in that proportion the disease is curable. They have only disappeared because newer ones have come up. It is quite a common thing for old symptoms to appear after the aggravation has come, and hence we see the symptoms disappearing in the reverse order of their coming. Those symptoms that are present subside, and old symptoms keep coming up. The physician must know himself that the patient is on the road to recovery, and it is well to say to the patient that this is encouraging; that diseases get well from above downwards, etc. Old symptoms often come back and go off without any change of medicine. It indicates that the medicine must be let alone. If the old symptoms come back to stay then a repetition of the dose is often necessary.

The twelfth observation. We will notice sometimes that *symptoms take the wrong direction.* For instance, if you prescribe for a rheumatism of the knees or feet, or for a rheumatism of the

hands, and relief takes place at once in the rheumatism of the
extremities, but the patient is taken down with violent internal
distress that settles in the region of the heart, or centres in the
spine, you see at once a transference has taken place from circumference to centre, and the remedy must be antidoted at once,
otherwise structural change will take place in that new site. When
diseases go from centre to circumference, going out from the
centres of life, out from the heart, lungs, brain and spine, out from
the interiors, upon the extremities, it is well. So it is that we find
most gouty patients get along best when their fingers and toes are
in the worst condition. To prescribe for this, and see the heart
symptoms grow worse is a most uncomfortable state of affairs, for
it is attended with a gradual downward tendency. Eruptions upon
the skin and affections in the extremities are good signs. I remember one time I was discharged from a violent old woman with
quite a considerable amount of Billingsgate, who told me that
when she called me in she could walk about, and now her ankles
were swelled up with rheumatism so that she could not move. That
patient got another doctor, but soon died. There is a great danger
in selecting a remedy on external symptoms alone, *i.e.*, selecting
a remedy that corresponds only to the skin and ignoring all the
symptoms that the patient may have, ignoring the whole economy
and general state of the patient; because it is true that that remedy
that is related to the skin alone may drive in that skin disease and
cause it to disappear while the patient himself is not cured. Such
a patient will remain sick until that eruption comes back again, or
locates in another place.

LECTURE XXXVI

THE SECOND PRESCRIPTION

The second prescription may be a repetition of the first, or it may be an antidote or a complement; but none of these things can be considered unless the record has been again fully studied, unless the first examination, and all the things that have since arisen, have been carefully restudied that they may be brought again to the mind of the physician. This is one of the difficulties to contend with when patients change doctors, and one of the reasons why patients do not do well after such a change. The strict homœopathic physician knows the importance of this and will try to ascertain the first prescription. If the former physician is strictly a homœopathic physician, he is most competent of all others to make the second prescription. It is often a hardship for a patient to fall into the hands of a second doctor, no matter how much Materia Medica he may know. The medicine that has partly cured the case can often finish it, and that medicine should not be changed until there are good reasons for changing it. It is a very common thing for patients to come to me from the hands of good prescribers. I tell them to stay with their own doctor. I do not want them. Such changing is often a detriment to the patient, unless he brings a full record, and this is especially true in relation to a case that has been partially cured, where the remedy has acted properly. If the patient has no reasonable excuse to leave the doctor, it is really a matter of detriment to the patient for a physician to take another's patients at such a moment. It is not so much a question of ethics, it is not so much a question of the relation of one doctor to another because friends can stand all that, but it is only after a tedious inspection of all the symptoms that an intelligent physician is capable of making a second prescription. As a general thing, if the first prescription has been beneficial it ought not to be left until it has done all that it can do. How is the second physician to know that? Then the duty of the physician is first to the patient, and to persuade the patient to return to his first doctor.

The rule is, after the first correction and homœopathic prescription, the striking features for which that remedy was administered

236   KENT'S LECTURES

have been removed, a change has come, and the guiding symptoms
of the case have been taken out, and only the common and trivial
symptoms remain. It is true if the physician would wait long
enough he would see the return of those symptoms, but usually
when a patient walks into a doctor's office the doctor is in a hurry
to make a prescription and does not wait until the proper time. He
at once prescribes on the symptoms that are left, and this is one
of the dangers to be avoided, a hurried second prescription. The
patients are to be pitied that fall into the hands of such homœopaths. Many patients are wonderfully benefited by the first prescription; they have said to me "Dr. So and So benefited me wonderfully for a while, and then he did not seem to be able to do me
any good." The fact was that the first prescription was a correct one,
having been properly chosen, and after that first prescription the
doctor administered his medicine so hastily and so indiscriminately
that nothing more was accomplished in the case. The trouble was
that he did not wait long enough. It makes no difference whether
the physician is so extremely conscientious that he does not want
to give Sac. Iac., or whether he is so ignorant that he does not
know how to give it, the result is the same. The early repetition of
the medicine and the continued giving of the same medicine, will
prevent anything like an opportunity for the making of a second
prescription.

If the doctor administers a well-chosen remedy, and repeats it
too soon, he never gives the symptoms a chance to come back and
call for a second prescription; but they come intermingled with
drug symptoms, so that the rational second prescription cannot be
made. The second prescription presupposes that the first one has
been a correct one, that it has acted, and that it has been let alone.
If the first prescription has not acted curatively, or has not been
permitted to act the full time, it is impossible to get a second
observation. The second observation is made when the case comes
to a standstill, for after the first prescription has been made changes
occur; there is a coming and going of symptoms, and while these
changes are occurring no rational observation can be made of the
case; if a second prescription be made during this time, it will be
likely to spoil the whole case. If the patient is not given a perfect
rest, if medicines are not kept out of the case, we will have no
opportunity to make a rational second prescription. But if these pre-
cautions are observed, then we can really make an observation

upon the return of the original symptoms, which is the first thing to be considered. Perhaps they are not so marked, but that is always the first thing to be looked for, the return of the original symptoms. While the confusion is going on after the administration of the remedy, while internal order is being established in the economy, we do not have the return of the original symptoms. This may be a matter of days, or weeks, or months, but if the return of symptoms is not observed what is there to be done?

Without symptoms what can the homœopathic physician do? No matter what state the patient is in, what can the physician do without symptoms? There is no earthly guide to the remedy except by signs and symptoms. So that it is the duty of the physician to *wait for the return of the original symptoms.* If the symptoms return somewhat as they were, differing slightly in their intensity, increased or decreased, it is good. If the patient has not had these present symptoms for some time, if there has been a relief caused by the first prescription, and then the symptoms return somewhat as in the original, this is one of the reasons for believing that the first prescription was a good one. If, after an interval of two or more months, the original symptoms return, we need very little information beyond this to know that the first prescription was a good one. In such a case when the symptoms return, when the patient has the same general and particulars as formerly, it means that the first prescription was a good one, that the case is curable, and that the second prescription must be a repetition of the former.

Another reason for making a second prescription is the appearance of a lot of new symptoms taking the place of the old symptoms; the old symptoms do not return, but new symptoms come in their place. The patient says: "Well, doctor, you have cured me of those symptoms I had, but now I have these." The doctor, after examining carefully these new symptoms, immediately looks up the pathogenesis, and it is possible that he will find these symptoms in the drug that he has administered and then it looks like a proving. He asks the patient if he ever had these symptoms before. "Never to my recollection, doctor." Cross-examine him carefully to see if he is not mistaken, until it seems that they are really new symptoms. If so, the remedy has not acted properly. It was not homœopathic to the case; and yet it was an unfortunate prescription, because it has caused the disease to progress in another direction, developing another group of symptoms.

This coming up of new symptoms means that they must be *antidoted*, if it is possible. The new symptoms combining with the old ones must be again studied and the second remedy must correspond more particularly to the new than to the old. It may cause the new symptoms to disappear and possibly have an effect upon the old ones. Any subsequent prescription takes into account all the things that have preceded it, all the conditions that have arisen, and, the third, fourth, fifth or sixth prescriptions have the same difficulties to surmount that are to be surmounted in the second. If the first prescription was an unfortunate one, then all the others are made with difficulty and fear.

It is rarely the case that a new prescription become necessary when the case merely comes to a standstill. The first prescription has been made and the symptoms commence to change in an orderly way; they change and interchange and new symptoms come up, but finally the symptoms go back to their original state, not marked enough to be of any importance, without any special suffering to the patient, and the patient has arrived at a state of standstill. The patient says, "I have no symptoms, yet I am not improving; I seemed to have come to a standstill position." He says this as to himself, not as to the symptoms. He has come to a standstill.

It is the duty of the physician then to wait, and wait a long time, but if after many months no outward symptoms have appeared, no external tendency of the disease, it is true that another dose of the same medicine will not do harm and the same remedy is the only one that can be considered. A new one cannot be entertained, because there is no guide to it; but another dose of the same medicine can cause the patient to be jogged along the way of feeling better, but there should never be any haste about it. Wait a long time when patients come to a standstill; but when, as in the first instance, the return of the original symptoms is observed, then you have some guide to the administration of the medicine.

The second prescription, then, technically speaking, is the prescription after the one that has acted. You may administer a dozen remedies without having any effect upon the economy, and yet no prescription has been administered that has been specific. You may fool away much time in administering remedies that are not related to the case. The result is the same. Consider the first prescription the one that has acted, that one has effected changes, and subsequent to that the next prescription is the second.

The next thing we have to consider *is the change of the remedy in a second prescription.* Under what circumstances must we change the remedy? One instance I have mentioned, when striking new symptoms appear, and there is an entire change of base in the symptoms, so that the headache, perhaps, which has lasted a long time, disappears. After the administration of the medicine, when a new group of symptoms appears somewhere in the body relative to the patient, such as the patient has never had, this new group of symptoms means that a new remedy must be considered, and under such circumstances the change of the remedy will be the second prescription, and the second prescription in this case calls for a change of remedy.

We will suppose another instance where the remedy must be changed. A patient has been for years under treatment for a constitutional chronic disorder, and you have gone through the potencies ranging from the lowest to the highest, and they have acted curatively. You have administered the different potencies, repeating the same potency until it would not act any longer, and then going higher, until you have gone through the whole range of potencies. You can repeat that remedy many times on a paucity of symptoms, when you cannot give another remedy, simply because it has demonstrated itself to be the patient's constitutional remedy. This remedy should not be changed so long as the curative action can be maintained. Even if the symptoms have been changed do not change the remedy, provided the patient has continuously improved. If the patient says he has improved continuously, and though it would be impossible for you, at this date, from the present symptoms, to select that remedy, hold on to that remedy, so long as you can secure improvement and good from it, though the symptoms have changed. Many physicians say: "If the symptoms change, I change the remedy." That is one of the most detrimental things that can be done. Change the remedy if the symptoms have changed, providing the patient has not improved; but if the patient has improved, though the symptoms have changed, continue that remedy so long as the patient improves. Very often the patients are giving forth symptoms long forgotten. The patient has not heard them, or has not felt them because he has become accustomed to them, like the ticking or the striking of the clock on the wall. Many of the symptoms that appear, and the slightest changes that occur, are old symptoms coming back. The patient is not always able to say that they are old symptoms returning, but finally the daughter or somebody in the house will delight you by saying that her mother had these things years ago and she has forgotten them. This is likely to be the case whenever a patient is proving. So long as curatve action can be obtained, and even though the symptoms have changed, provided the patient is improving, hands off. Whenever in doubt, wait. It is a rule after you have gone through a series of potencies, never to leave that remedy until one or more dose of a higher potency has been given and tested. But when this dose of a higher potency has been given and tested, without effect, that is the only means you have of knowing that this remedy has done all the good it can for this patient and that a change is necessary.

There is another instance to be spoken of, and that is when the second prescription becomes a complementary one. A second prescription is sometimes necessary to complement the former and this is always a change of remedy. Suppose a little four or five year old child, a large-headed, bright, blue-eyed boy, is subject to taking cold, and every cold settles in the head with flushed face and throbbing carotids, etc., you say give him *Belladonna* and *Bell.* relieves, but it does not act as a constitutional remedy. He continues to have these headaches, which are due to a psoric constitution, and the time comes when *Bell.* will not relieve them; but upon a thorough study of the case, you find that when his symptoms are not acute, when he does not have this cold and fever, he does not have the headache and you see an entirely different remedy indicated. You study over the flabby muscles, and you find his glands are enlarged; that he takes cold with every change in the weather, like enough he craves eggs, and you decide that the case calls for *Calcarea.* The fact that *Bell.* was so closely related to him and only acted as a palliative further emphasizes it. It is a loss of time to treat more than the first or second acute paroxysm. Do not give *Calcarea* during the paroxysm, but after the wire edge has been rubbed off by *Bell.*, give him that constitutional remedy that is complementary to *Bell.*, which is *Calcarea.* Many remedies associate after this fashion.

Then there are series of remedies, as, for instance, *Sulphur, Calcarea* and *Lycopodium.* A medicine always leads to one of its own cognates, and we find that the cognates are closely related to each other, like *Sepia* and *Nux Vomica*. A bilious fever in a *Sepia* constitution is likely to call for *Nux*, and as soon as that bilious fever or remittent fever has subsided the symptoms of *Sepia* come out immediately, showing the complementary relation of *Nux* and *Sepia*. If the patient has been under the influence of *Sepia* some time, and comes down with some acute inflammatory attack, he is very likely to run towards *Nux* or another of its cognates. The whole Materia Medica abounds with these complementary and cognate relationships.

The second prescription also takes into consideration the change of plan of treatment. The plan of treatment consists in assuming that the case is a psoric one, if looming up before the eyes, all the symptoms in the case and its history indicate psora. The treatment has probably consisted of *Sulphur*, *Graphites* and such medicines as are well-known to be anti-psorics. The symptoms have run to these remedies; but, behold, after you have made the patient wonderfully well, and you have effected marked changes in his system, so that the psoric symptoms have disappeared, he comes into your office with an ulcerated sore throat, with dreadful head pains and with the constitutional state and appearance that will lead you to say, "My dear sir, did you ever have syphilis?" "Yes, twenty or thirty years ago, and it was cured with Mercury." Now, the psoric condition has been subdued and this old syphilitic condition has come up. This, then indicates a second prescription. You have to adjust your remedies to an entirely new state of things. So it is also with regard to sycosis; these states may alternate with each other. When one is uppermost, the other is quiet, so you have to change your plan of treatment according to the state of the patient.

No prescription can be made for any patient except after a careful and prolonged study of the case, to know what it promises in the symptoms, and everything that has existed previously. That is the important thing. Always restudy your cases. Do not administer a medicine without knowing the constitution of the patient, because it is a hazardous and dangerous thing to do.

LECTURE XXXVII

DIFFICULT AND INCURABLE CASES—PALLIATION

While Homœopathy itself is a perfect science, its truth is only partially known. The truth itself relates to the Divine, the knowledge relates to man. It will require a long time before physicians become genuine masters in this truth. In Switzerland the children have been raised for centuries to the knowledge that it is necessary to make watches perfectly, they have been raised, as it were, in the watch factories. Now, when Homœopathy is hundreds of years old, and little ones grow up into the knowledge of it and observe and practise it, our successors will acquire knowledge that we do not possess now. Things will grow brighter as minds are brought together and men think harmoniously. The more we keep together the better, and the more we think as one the beter. It is a pity that differences should arise among us when we have so perfect a truth to bind us together.

It is very rarely the case that among the provings of our remedies not one is to be found which corresponds to the characteristic features of a case. It was rarely so in Hahnemann's day, and it is certainly very rarely the case with our voluminous Materia Medica. Beginners, of course, are obliged to rely very largely upon the repertories. This one thing you can depend upon, the image of the patient's illness becomes more simple when you have done your best to prescribe one remedy after another. In these difficult cases, when you have zigzagged the patient for a number of years, you will find his symptoms become more definite and striking and more clearly understood. Sometimes when I have worked patiently upon a patient for a long time, and I have given several remedies, and the patient has partially improved, she has become disappointed and run off to somebody else, but would come back again and say I had done more for her than anyone else and she would try again. I have found in such instances that time has done much, and that I had little trouble then to grasp the case and make rapid progress. In addition to that, she comes back with a patient state of mind, which is more helpful to the physician than to her. The confidence of the patient helps the physician to find the right remedy. His mind works much better when he feels he is trusted; the confidence of the patient sharpens his intelligence.

Closely analogous to these cases are what may be called alternating complaints and one-sided complaints, those that show but one side. It is not uncommon for a patient's malady to have two sides —one side being manifested when the other side is not. Eye symptoms may be present when the stomach symptoms are absent. You may find that Euphrasia is more sharply related to the eye symptoms than the antipsoric that fits the whole case, and that Pulsatilla fits the stomach symptoms much better than the antipsoric that fits the whole case, but remember that there is one antipsoric that is more similar to the whole patient than these special remedies, because it is better fitted to the generals. The oftener you prescribe for different groups of symptoms the worse it is for your patient, because it tends to rivet the constitutional state upon the patient and to make him incurable. Do not prescribe until you have found the remedy that is similar to the whole case, even although it is clear in your mind that one remedy may be more similar to one particular group of symptoms and another remedy to another group. Very often a remedy that will go to the very centre and restore order to the economy will cause quite a turmoil. These alternating and one-sided complaints are sometimes dreadful to manage, and when everything is thrown to the surface or the extremities, e.g., when gouty and rheumatic symptoms have an outward tendency, the patient will run off and leave you.

Incurable complaints—and you meet many will trouble any physician. The allopath has the means of putting the patients under the influence of strong drugs and making them imagine that something is being done to their benefit, whereas injury is being done whenever they are patched up by strong drugs. It is unaccountable, therefore, that some of our homœopathic practitioners make use of palliatives that are so detrimental to the patient.

The physician who applies the single remedy in potentized form under the Law of Cure any length of time will easily be convinced that there is no other way of palliation that holds out any permanent hope for the patient. Opium will sometimes relieve pain, stop diarrhœa, and mitigate cough, but woe to the patient. It so annuls reaction that there is no possible development of the symptoms that are necessary to indicate what homœopathic remedy the patient needs, and while the pain is stopped the patient is not cured. What has been said of Opium is as true of all drugs given to relieve pain. When an opiate must be given, let it be clearly understood that a cure of this patient is abandoned. What thoughtful physician will abandon the hope of a cure during painful sicknesses so long as life endures. In consumption and cancer and wasting sickness the remedy that is most similar to the painful groups of symptoms will ever give the most relief and it is a forlorn hope that tempts its abandonment.